ACUPUNCTURE TECHNIQUES 102

Moxibustion, Three-Edged Needle, Cutaneous Needle Therapy, Gua Sha, Cupping, and Electroacupuncture

By Cat Calhoun, MAcOM, L.Ac.

Cats TCM Notes Press
San Miguel de Allende, Mexico

Acupuncture Techniques 102 - Acknowledgments

For DeLora, a fellow healer.
I couldn't ask for a better partner on the path.

ACKNOWLEDGMENTS

No one does anything truly on one's own. I thought myself totally self-sufficient before I dove into the study of Chinese medicine. When that journey began, my eyes opened to the myriads of those who were actively helping me, those who have gone before, and even those who will come long after I'm gone. We are interconnected. You are me, I am you.

I especially want to thank Dr. Linda Yuxia Qiu, my acupuncture techniques professor, an amazing medical Qigong practitioner, and quite possibly a Daoist immortal in disguise. Thank you for subtly pointing the way to "more." Thank you too, to Dr. Xiaotian Shen, one of my favorite clinical supervisors, for the hands-on teaching and cool clinical pearls you dropped for me along the way.

Thank you to Lisa Lapwing, a most awesome practitioner based in Orlando Florida. We studied together, practiced together, we practiced *on* each other in student clinic, and then we became each other's practitioners! Not having Lisa in my daily life is my one giant regret about moving to Mexico.

Thank you to my buds: Donna "Needles" Tatum, Tiffany Chiu Peralez, Vanessa Olsen, Andi Kohn, Mark Hernandez, and Katherine Webster. To Georgie Hoiseth, a kick ass practitioner and fellow computer geek, I thank thee! To Rita Ramirez, I would *not* want to be on this journey without you!

To my patients, whom I learn from every day and who trust me with state of their health, thank you. I love having you in my life.

And to so many more who have loved, supported, and believed in me, I express my gratitude and thanks. May the deity of your choice look favorably upon you all!

Cat Calhoun, MsAcOM, L.Ac

INTRODUCTION

Chinese Medicine practitioners do way more than just acupuncture. If you've been to an acupuncturist you may have experienced cupping, gua sha, moxibustion (often referred to simply as 'moxa'), e-stim, microcurrent, bleeding techniques, sound healing, breath work, Chinese massage (tuina), meditation instruction, and more.

Some of these techniques you will pick up on your own later, but as part of your foundational education, you do need to learn the basics for these modalities:

- Moxibustion (moxa)
- Three-edged needle technique (bleeding therapy)
- Cutaneous needle therapy
- Gua sha
- Cupping
- Electroacupuncture (EA or e-stim)

This page intentionally left blank.

Acupuncture Techniques 102 - Introduction

TABLE OF CONTENTS

This page intentionally left blank.

SECTION 1
Moxibustion

Moxibustion is the burning of materials on or near the skin for therapeutic benefit to the patient. Generally this material is *Artemisia vulgaris*, but that can vary.

This section covers materials used for moxibustion (often nicknamed "moxa"), safety concerns, methods of use for some of the wide variety of moxa materials, precautions and contraindications.

A cautionary note about moxibustion

One thing to note about moxibustion: the most common method is the use of the herb Artemis vulgaris. When burned this herb smells a *lot* like marijuana smoke. It also clings to your clothes and skin, so it can smell like you've been partying like a fool rather than healing people.

Caution #1

This can be a concern to your business neighbors when you have your own clinic. I've had several business owners come storming out of their offices to ask who was lighting up. I learned quickly to introduce myself to surrounding businesses when I am practicing in a new clinic space, explain what I do and what they might smell.

If there is tremendous concern, I generally use smokeless moxa (which I don't love, but whatever), or combine spray-on moxa with the use of a heat lamp instead.

Caution #2

If you have kids, be aware that when you use regular moxibustion materials you will smell like you've been smoking enormous amounts of pot.

I have known several practitioners who were not allowed to pick up their kids at school, who had child protective services called on them, and more because teachers or neighbors just didn't understand what they did for a living and what that entailed.

CHAPTER 1
Introduction to Moxibustion

MULTI-CULTURAL MOXA

Moxibustion, often just called "moxa" among us acupuncture geeks, is an extremely old technique, recorded very early in written history. It probably comes from more northern areas of the world where the temperatures are colder and cold animals like dairy would have exacerbated digestive difficulties and coldness in the limbs.

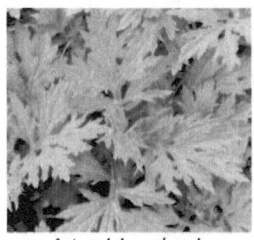

Artemisia vulgaris

Moxa comes from an herb that is also called "mugwort" in western herbal traditions. Mugwort is commonly known as *Artemisia vulgaris*, though in Japanese herbal traditions, the variety *A. princeps* (or *A. indica*) is more commonly used.

Mugwort has been used for thousands of years in both western and eastern herbalism. The taxonomic name, *A. vulgaris,* is named after the Goddess Artemis,[1] goddess of the moon. In western herbal traditions it is often used in teas or tinctures to treat women's diseases such as irregular and painful periods, PMS, and endometriosis. It's also used as a calmative for difficult emotions like anxiousness, stress, tension, and insomnia. It's also used as an antidepressant in combination with other herbs as well.[2]

If you look into Asian herbal medicine you will also find herb in use in Japan, China, Tibet, Mongolia, and India. In Chinese medicine it is considered to be a blood mover. The internal form

---

[1] https://gingerwebb.com/mm-mugwort/
[2] https://www.youtube.com/watch?v=9weSiB7qLJE

of the herb is called Ai Ye and is used to treat women's diseases, mostly that stem from cold influences, much like it is in western herbal traditions. It also dispels damp and cold and moves blood and Qi.

What we are going to do with it in this book is burn it on the exterior of the body. That's when it becomes moxa rather than ai ye!

Moxa that is processed for burning on the exterior of the body is called "moxa wool." Moxa wool is burned either directly on the skin or held just above the skin as it burns (called 'indirect moxa' to heat the points you want to treat. Other herbs can be combined with moxa such as ginger or garlic to get different therapeutic effects. We will cover some of those other herbs in this chapter.

When moxa is burned on or near the skin, it warms the meridians and dispels cold from them. It also moves Qi and Blood to open the meridians for proper flow.

COMMON MOXA MATERIALS

Moxibustion is a popular and effective therapy, so it is sold in a rather astonishing array of forms. We will cover the most common ones here, but be aware that it *is* sold in a crazy wide variety of application forms.

Loose Moxa

The go-to form for most acupuncture students and for a lot of practitioners is the light, fluffy loose moxa wool. You will use loose moxa to form cones of various sizes to burn on the skin surface and you will use it to create a small wad that is then placed on the top of an acupuncture needle for 'warm needle therapy.' They can also be used with some moxa boxes.

Get good quality moxa wool. It should be loose and fluffy. The highest quality types are a bluish yellow in color. If you find moxa wool that has already turned a darker olive green, it's not fresh. Buy the quality bluish yellow stuff and keep it in a cool dry place. It will keep for a couple of years this way.

Here's a comparison chart of good quality moxa and poor quality moxa.

High Quality	Poor Quality
Old/aged	Newly harvested
Bluish yellow color	Darker – brownish to black
Fine, like wool	Thicker fibers
Pure - no other stuff in it	Impure, other fibers mixed in
Soft to the touch, fluffy	Resistant, harder
Dry	Wet to moist
Burns smoothly	Have to relight it a lot
Forms cones easily	Hard to roll cones

Moxa Sticks

These are pre-rolled sticks of moxa wool. There are both pure moxa and moxa+herb mixes of these sticks. You can find most good moxa sticks rolled into a mulberry paper. Some of these are mixed with a type of musk that helps with penetration of the moxa into the channel.

Smokeless moxa sticks

I love/hate these. Moxa smoke is the most challenging thing about using moxa, so these can be a good alternative if you have ventilation issues in your clinic space. *But* they have a lot of chemical elements to them that are not so desirable. Use them if you absolutely must, but be aware of this.

Stick-on moxa

These are mini-moxa devices with a little bit of sticky on the bottom so you can attach them to various locations and burn them as you would a cone. Personally, I prefer the cones, but they are pretty handy for getting moxa, needles, and other forms of treatment all in a single one-hour patient session.

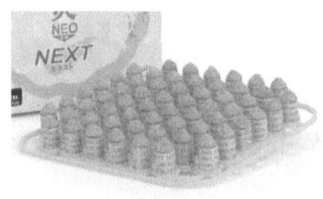

Moxa caps

Moxa caps go on top of a needle for warm needle therapy. Yes, you could roll a small wad of it and pop it on top of any needle you want, but the moxa caps can be very handy because they are so easy to use. They also come in a smokeless variety if that's what you need.

Moxa Spray

I have to confess, I love this stuff. This is literally a spray-on form of moxa, but also comes in roll-ons and creams. I don't find it to be as effective as burning moxa, but does work well if you apply a heat lamp over the treated area.

MOXIBUSTION "GEAR" WORTH MENTIONING

There is a crazy array of "gear" you can get for moxibustion application and use. You can go completely nutso buying it, but resist temptation until you can write it off later as a business expense!

Gear	What it's used for and why you might want it
Trays and saucers	Though there are all kinds of things you could use, I recommend these, especially while you are in school. These are light weight and durable. • Tray to hold your cones. I use a small open tray like you would use in an autoclave. Light weight, sterilizable, multi-use.

Gear	What it's used for and why you might want it
	• Needle saucer. I like these because of the "scoop" lip on one end. Super easy to put this edge right next to the burning moxa cone and scoop the cone off while pushing on the other side with forceps.
Jar with lid	Small to medium glass jar with a lid. Fill it about ½ full with water and place the spent moxa cones in here (lit side down) and cover to minimize smell and safely extinguish burning cones. Wrap it in bubble wrap if you are carrying it around in your pack. By the way, I used a plastic cup for a while because I broke my jar, but one of the cones bumped up against the wall of it and burned a hole through it. That was a mess.
Forceps	I use these to scoop the spent moxa off onto the needle tray or directly into the glass jar. Depends on how well that cone held together and how far down it burned.
Extinguisher	These are used to both hold and extinguish burning moxa sticks. I recommend the type that is mounted into a bowl that also catches the ash.
Moxa burners	Lots of varieties of these. I'll cover some of the most basic types, but know that there are tons of variations. • Tiger and Lion warmers Both hold moxa sticks. The tiger warmer allows you to adjust the level of heat and keep your hand safe while moving the stick over the surface of the skin. Lion warmers can

Gear	What it's used for and why you might want it
	roll on the surface of the skin • Moxa boxes. You'll find these in many configurations from large ones that sit on bigger body surfaces (lower back, lower abdomen, etc) to small hand-held to "bowls" that hold multiple sticks. There is a fun link to a Youtube video below where you can see one of these in action.[3]
Spoon or scoop for moxa caps	These fun devices scoop and catch the ash for moxa (balls or caps) you've placed on the top of needles for warm needle therapy. These devices have a slot you slide over the needle. The larger of the two in the graphic can scoop and hold more than one burning moxa cap at a time.
Index cards and scissors	My professors used these to put at the base of any needle we were using with warm needle therapy. This catches the ash so you don't burn your patient. This reduces your liability. You still have to watch carefully when you do moxibustion regardless of how many safety procedures you have in place, but this helps.
Burn cream	We refer to this as "miracle Chinese burn cream" in my house . Great for burns, scrapes, and bites. Pretty miraculous stuff. There are a number of types you can get, but this is my fave. Technically this is called Ching Wan Hung. You can

---

[3] https://youtu.be/Pp0XFPGa7PE?t=43

Gear	What it's used for and why you might want it
	get it on Amazon, LhasaOMS, and other places.
Incense gear	You need lightly scented incense sticks and a sturdy base that is easy to get the stick in and out of and that has a good ash catcher. There are some very good Japanese stick incenses that work well for this.
Candle gear	It's so much easier to light the incense with a candle in a holder with a good sturdy base than it is to use a lighter. A votive candle works just fine for this. You can also use the candle later when you do fire twinkling cupping.

FUNCTIONS AND INDICATIONS OF MOXA

So what all do we use moxibustion for anyway? Here are the biggies.

Function	Indications and Discussion
Warms meridians, expels wind, cold, damp	• Wind cold and wind damp cold invasions Moxa at Du 14 for example • Internal cold symptoms Example: live in a cold area and frequently feel cold in the spine. You could use it at Du 4 and Ren 4 to warm the body and the channels. • Yang deficiencies I.e., Sp yang xu – frequent cold, diarrhea, want to eat warm foods/drinks. Use at Sp points • Bi Syndromes due to wind, damp and cold. Bi syndromes are pain syndromes – usually they refer to arthritis. You can warm local arthritis points that are sensitive to cold with moxa.

Function	Indications and Discussion
Regulates Qi and Blood	Qi and Blood problems of all kinds. Examples: • Pain and numbness on the skin due to poor blood or Qi flow. Moxa in the local area to improve flow of both Qi and Blood. • Qi sinking. Use moxa at Du 20 to lift the Qi. • Liver Yang Rising. Use moxa at Kidney 1 to direct the Qi downward. • Use it to stimulate points instead of using needles. You will find in some Asian medicine schools that moxa is used more than just it's herbal applications. It is used to stimulate points all over the body by burning small rice-grain sized moxa cones rather than inserting needles. This is fairly common in Japanese acupuncture for example.
Revive Yang	Used in Yang Collapse Syndrome to revive Yang. Use a fu zi cake and burn the cone on top of that for this purpose.
Prevent disease and maintain health	In Chinese medicine, this generally refers to "scarring moxa." In Japanese medicine very small moxa cones are used for this in a non-scarring manner In scarring moxa, small moxa cones are burned on St 36 regularly to the point that they blister. This stimulates the body to boost the immune system and functions as kind of an immune booster. Some people do this before traveling to a different climate and may patients over the age of 60 in China will have this done regularly to maintain health. *But,* don't do this to young people! Young

Function	Indications and Discussion
	people have a higher level of Yang already and this can create too much heat in their bodies.
Dissipate nodules, remove toxic heat	You can do this at the early stage of a sore, boil, or carbuncle *before* the pus forms. Use an indirect moxa - burn a cone on top of a thin slice of garlic with a holes poked in it to let the heat through for this. Works as a kind of local antibiotic. It's also been used with scrofula in the same manner as well as sores, boils, and carbuncles that have persisted for a very long tie and won't heal. This signals an immunity weakness and the indirect moxa + garlic gives both the "antibiotic" effect and a boost to the immune system.

This page intentionally left blank.

CHAPTER 2
Methods of Moxibustion Application

Moxibustion can be applied either directly to the skin (direct moxa), or indirectly. Indirect moxa could be held over the surface of the skin in a variety of ways or it can mean you are applying a moxa cone to the skin with a layer of something else between the burning cone and the skin.

Acupuncture Techniques classes, no matter what they are called in your school, are very hands-on, "doing-based" classes. You cannot learn everything you need to know from a book. You need your professor's expertise and finesse.

So with that in mind, let's get to it.

DIRECT MOXIBUSTION

In direct moxibustion, a cone of moxa is applied directly to the skin, often with a very thin layer of burn cream on the surface of the skin.

Moxibustion materials are rolled into cones in various sizes for different applications and areas of the body. In Chinese medicine the cones are generally one of three sizes.

Small	About the size of wheat kernel
Medium	About the size of a bean
Large	About ½ the size of an olive

In Japanese acupuncture, the smallest moxa cones are about the size of a grain of rice – even smaller than above. I can roll the Chinese sizes but have a very hard time with the tiny rice grain moxa! Those take a ton of practice.

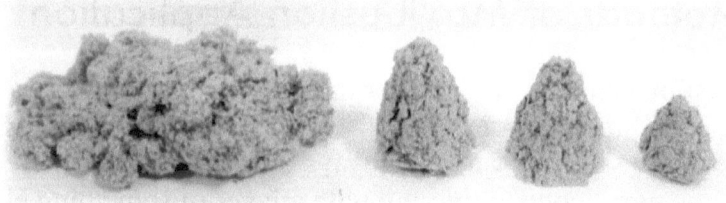

Learning exercise

Practicing rolling various sizes of moxa cones. Your instructor will guide you in this. Make sure you can roll any size as needed and that the process becomes automatic and easy. You can keep practicing with the same bundle of moxa, making and unmaking these cones as often as you need to.

Clinical application of direct moxibustion

Any moxibustion in which the moxa comes into contact with the skin and is burned on the skin is direct moxibustion. Direct moxa can be non-scarring and scarring .

Non-scarring moxa

Non-scarring moxa is often applied for chronic cold deficiencies, skin warts, and for general health maintenance. Non-scarring moxa is done as follows. For now, stick with burning one cone at one location at a time.

1. Gather your materials and accessories, roll the appropriate number and size of cones, and get your tools ready, including your jar of water with lid. Fill the jar about ½ full.

2. Verify that you have a signed informed consent form and that you have told the patient what this procedure entails. This includes telling them exactly what's going to happen and what they might expect to feel during the process. . . including the marijuana smell that isn't really marijuana.

3. Apply a very thin layer of burn cream to the site or sites in which you will burn the moxa cones.

4. Place a cone on the point and on top of the burn cream.

5. Tell the patient you are about to light the cone and to tell you as soon as they feel the warmth of the cone *and* then tell you as soon as it begins to feel too intense.

6. Use the glowing tip of your incense stick to light the tip of the moxa cone. Immediately place the incense back into the holder and get your needle tray and forceps ready.

7. The patient will tell you when they can first feel the warmth of the lit cone. Be ready to remove the cone. Shortly thereafter, they should tell you when it's starting to feel too intense.

8. Remove the smoldering cone immediately.

    I scoop under the cone with the lip of the needle saucer on one side and push toward that lip with the forceps on the other side. Drop the burning one, lit side down into the jar with water in it.

Put the lid on the jar.

9. Repeat steps 3 through 7 as needed.

10. When you are done, you need to clean up the sites you used. I blot away the burn cream and any moxa crumbs with a soft paper towel. I recommend the Viva towels if you can find them. They are the softest disposable towels I've found.

Scarring moxa

I'm not even gonna lie: in all my years in both student clinic and then running my own practice for more than a decade, *not one person* has agreed to scarring moxa – neither fellow students, nor patients. It was mentioned and described, but never actually taught in my classes. I've only seen a video or two on it, so I don't really feel qualified to speak much about it.

Check this video out. If you practice in the United States maybe this will give you an idea why it is not actively encouraged in our extremely litigious and pain-averse society, even though it has amazing benefits. (Some of those include successful treatment of asthma, chronic fatigue syndrome, chronic gastritis, and weakened constitutions.)

https://www.youtube.com/watch?v=PMzpxv3C5Dw

Also, caution patients to avoid heavy work and to keep the blister and local area clean to avoid infection.

Two unusual direct moxa applications

- Rush burning moxa
  It isn't Artemisia that is used for this procedure, but an herb called deng xin cao. Deng xin cao is a rush (the herb, not rush as in 'omigod I'm in a hurry' or 'wow! what a ride!'). It looks like dry rice noodles, but it's a plant.

  This bit of rush is soaked in oil, lit on one end and then touched to a point to create a little brown spot/scar. This can treat mumps, but again is pretty rare to see in the western world.

- Crude herb moxa
  This method uses fresh Artemisia rather than dried and processed to create a small blister on the point that gives benefits like that of scarring moxa. This can be used for chronic asthma which has its' root in Yang Qi xu and phlegm retention.

  On hot days the Yang Qi is natively stronger in the body because the environment supports the internal supply. Many asthma patients don't have active s/sx at this time. This is the time of the year in which it is best to treat asthma, especially to resolve deep stuck phlegm. Bladder 13, 20, and 43 are good for this moxa scar. The procedure is generally repeated three times in successive days.

Indirect moxa is any application of moxa that doesn't immediately touch the skin. This can be a moxa cone ontop of a buffer medium, warm needle therapy, use of moxa sticks above the surface of the skin, moxa boxes, and more.

Indirect moxibustion with a buffer medium

This method of moxa uses a buffer medium sitting on the skin and a moxibustion cone sitting on top of the buffer.

Ginger, garlic, salt, and fu zi cakes are the most commonly used herb buffers.

Buffer medium	When/how used
Ginger	Indications: • Expels cold • Releases exterior • Warms interior • Stops vomiting Moxa on ginger combines the action of the point you are using, of the heat, and of the ginger. Moxa is penetrating and pushes the action of the ginger into the point. You might use this for common cold, cough, wind damp Bi, vomiting, abdominal pain, diarrhea due to cold retention, wind cold damp Bi syndromes (think arthritis), Spleen or Kidney Yang xu, and more. How to: • Cut a slice of fresh ginger about .6 mm or ¼" thick. • Puncture holes in the ginger slice so that the moxa and heat can penetrate through it more easily. • Burn medium to large sized moxa

Buffer medium	When/how used
	cones on top of the ginger slice. You generally use 3-7 cones. You burn them until the patient says the area feels warm or until the skin is moist and reddish.
Garlic	Indications: • Removes toxins • Kills germs • Treats early stage carbuncles, sores, boils; also insect bites, psoriasis, tuberculosis, scrofula and more. This was a very common practice in China for tuberculosis. It was/is used on points related to Lungs, points to nourish Yin such as Bladder 13, Bladder 17, Bladder 19 (Bladder 17 and 19 are called the "Four Flowers" - nourish yin and blood to treat wasting that comes with TB). This method is also used for psoriasis at the local area affected. How to: The method for use is like the ginger slice steps listed above.

Salt	Indications:
	• Treats whole body problems
	Esp good for kids, but also for adults. Used at Ren 8, the portal we were all fed through for 9 months. This point is still a portal for transferring warmth and Qi. Can treat digestive, urinary, and reproductive system disorders.
	• Warms the interior
	    o Abdominal pain, umbilical area pain due to cold (shi or xu)
	    o Hernia pain – due to cold or acute onset.
	    o Prolonged dysentery or chronic

Buffer medium	When/how used
	diarrhea ○ Urinary retention (indicating chronic Kidney deficiency, prostate problems. Post surgical patients have this too, as surgery disturbs the local function). This also applies to patients with postpartum urinary retention. • Yang collapse S/sx: profuse cold sweating, cold extremities, hidden pulse. You could also use moxa by itself, but with salt is more effective. Now it is only used for severe yang deficiency. Not a convenient method basically, so modern method developed from this is a belt with a bag that can cover above abdomen so that the patient wears it. They can control the heat, turn on/off, etc. Similar effect. How to: In brief, you fill the umbilicus with salt and burn the moxa cone on top of it. But now the patient has a belly button full of salt and that's just annoying and messy. One of my professors suggested this: • Make a small paper cone out of a bit of paper towel that fits in the umbilicus. • Put the salt into the cone. • Place the moxa cone on top of the salt and light it with an incense stick. You can also place a slice of ginger on top of the salt and then the moxa cone on top of that. You can use other herbs too such as gui zhi (cinnamon twigs - warms the limbs well) or the white part of a green onion smashed into a pulp (good for urinary retention), etc.

Buffer medium	When/how used
	But, do not use garlic! Has some negative effects here. Don't do it.
Fu zi cake	Indications: • Warms the Kidney yang Yang xu sx such as impotence, premature ejaculation. Fu Zi is very hot/warm in nature, slightly toxic and requires some specific prep before you can take it *internally*. The processed fu zi cake, however, is safe. • Yin type sores These are long term, won't heal, pale color, not hot to touch, very little pain in local area. Indicates there is not enough Yang Qi to heal. Fu zi moxa will bring the Yang Qi back and help heal.

Indirect warm needle moxibustion

This combines acupuncture with moxibustion. This also warms and opens the channels and moves Qi and Blood.

To use this method you needle the point with a metal handled needle, get the qi, then put a wad of moxa wool on the handle of the needle. There are also pre-made compressed moxa caps you can buy to put on the top of the handle as well. Both work well, though I have a slight preference for the moxa wool.

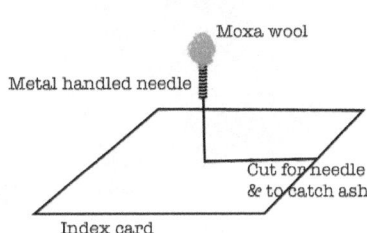

Moxa wool

Metal handled needle

Cut for needle & to catch ash

Index card

Dr. Qianzhi Wu, one of my clinic supervisors, would cut a square of index card about 2"x 2" (50mm^2) or a little bigger, then cut a slit in it from the center to one edge. He would then place the card under the moxa cone before lighting it to catch the falling ash.

This method still warms and opens the meridians and also moves Qi and Blood even though it's waaaay up on the handle of the needle and transfers the heat deeply into the body.

Indications:
Mainly used in local areas.
- Cold damp Bi syndromes with joint pain, numbness and cold sensations.
- Paralysis, muscle weakness and atrophy.

Use a scoop or moxa spoon to remove the spent wad of moxa or the moxa cap. This keeps both your hands and your patient safe from falling ash and burning materials.

Indirect moxibustion with a moxa box

A moxa box is a container with holes or screen in the bottom of the box. You put several moxa cones or sticks inside, light them, then put the lid back on. Use moxa boxes where the body will support the box like the lower abdomen or on the back. You put these in places where strong heat is needed.

These are generally places you would use to tonify Yang and Qi deficiencies. Heat helps to tonify Qi as well as Yang.

Never put a moxa box on the chest or upper back! Heat rises in the body just as it does in the environment and will put too much heat into the upper body causing insomnia, palpitations, and irritability.

Note: There are some moxa boxes that come with elastic straps and use moxa sticks instead of moxa cones that are fixed into the box. Some of these are suitable for use on the limbs.

If you want to see one of these in use, look at this Youtube video.
https://youtu.be/Pp0XFPGa7PE?t=43

Indirect moxibustion with moxa sticks

Moxa sticks are compressed rolls of moxa that come in a couple of varieties as discussed in the previous chapter. A moxa stick is used by the practitioner or the patient for 10-20 minutes over the site of treatment to get the desired effect.

I say "or the patient" because these are often used for chronic conditions. Acupuncturists will often teach a patient how to use the sticks and send them home with a couple of them as "homework" to extend the therapeutic effect of their treatments.

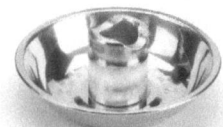 To use moxa sticks, get your materials together. You will need your moxa snuffer/holder, a lit candle, and the moxa stick itself. Have burn cream ready for those "uh oh" moments. Remember to roll the tip of the moxa stick frequently in your snuffer to get the ash off. Hot ash falling onto the skin is a quick way to really make a patient unhappy.

Moxa sticks are used in a variety of ways, depending on the therapeutic effect you want.

Method	Effect
Single point	In this method you hold the stick ½ to 1 inch over a specific point until the skin turns pink and warm. Adjust the height as needed so that the patient does not feel burned or uncomfortable. This stimulates the point in much the same way an acupuncture needle would.
Over an area	Move the stick at a slow to medium speed in a larger area than a single point. Circular motions over the affected areas such as painful joints work well. Hover over the surface of the skin ½ to 1 or more inches as needed. Be sensitive to the patient's pain tolerance and comfort levels.

You can also move the lit stick up and down an acupuncture channel to stimulate the channel and move/regulate Qi and Blood flow in that channel |
| Sparrow Pecking method | In this method you are slowly and repeatedly moving the lit end of the stick close to a point and then away from it. These warm/cool/warm/cool cycles are often more comfortable for the patient than holding the stick in place over a point and give similar benefits. |

Another moxa stick use I should mention is the use of a "tiger" or "lion" warmer.

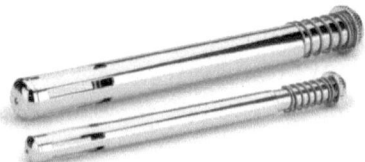

Tiger warmers hold the lit moxa stick inside the device. The distance from the lit tip to the metal point can be adjusted to get the level of heat you want. You can then place the tip of the tiger warmer against the skin to stimulate points. This can be very effective in areas where it is difficult to safely do direct moxa with cones, such as at Du 20, Yintang, and Taiyang areas.

Lion warmers look very similar, but can be rolled over the surface of the skin.

ORDER OF APPLICATION AND USE BASICS

The sensation on the skin when moxibustion is applies is generally a local warming sensation at first, then goes deeper inside and is often felt along the channel.

There is a recommended basic order to how you apply moxibustion and it is similar to the suggested order for acupuncture. Here are the general rules.

Order	Discussion
Posterior side 1st, anterior side 2nd.	The posterior side of the body, the back, is the Yang side. The Yang side is generally done first when applying moxibustion. Do that part of the treatment at the beginning, then have the patient turn over and do moxa on the Yin (anterior) side of the body.
Upper body 1st, lower body 2nd	This is the same idea as above – the upper body is relatively more Yang than the lower. Do moxa on the head, then body, then four limbs. You obviously won't do all of these points at the same time in the same treatment…

Order	Discussion
Smaller cones 1st, larger cones 2nd	Usually start with small and medium sized cones. The tiny ones are actually harder to control, so do it when your fingers are fresher. Be aware that larger cones might generate too much heat for your patient, so start smaller then see if their body needs bigger cones.
Fewer/smaller cones 1st, more cones later	Like with acupuncture, and especially with patients who haven't had moxa at all or have had it very little, start with a smaller amount and smaller cones. If their body requires more, you can roll bigger cones in successive treatments.

Commonly Used Points

There are some points that get a lot of moxa attention because they work so well with this method of treatment. The most common to use are:

Point	Some of the indications with moxa
Stomach 36	Tonifies Spleen and Stomach Qi, boosts the whole body and immune system
Ren 8	Tonifies, warms the whole body, moves Qi and blood. Abdominal pain, pain around the umbilicus, hernia pain, prolonged dysentery, chronic diarrhea, urinary retention and more.
Ren 4, 6	Tonifies Yuan Qi, Yang Qi, Kidney Qi
Ren 12	Nourishes Spleen and Stomach functions
Du 20, 14, 4	Lifts the Yang Qi of the whole body, especially of the Kidney
Bladder 23 and back shu points	Used to tonify the Zang organs

Point	Some of the indications with moxa
Kidney 1	Treats Yang rising, helps anchor it and bring it back down.
Spleen 1	Heavy menstruation
Bl 67	Helps turn a fetus that is not facing properly for birth.

Tonification and Reductions Methods Using Moxibustion

Method	Reduction or Tonification
Cones	**To reduce:** After you light it, blow on it so that the cone burns faster and the heat is more intense. **To tonify:** Let it burn naturally and extinguish on its' own (unless the heat starts feeling too intense to the patient, then scoop it off).
Monks' hood	This refers to indirect moxa on a fu zi cake – the other name for it is monk's hood. Fu zi always tonifies and strengthens the Yang.
Garlic	This refers to indirect moxa on a slice of garlic. Garlic removes toxins, so it always reduces.
Area	The area upon which you use moxa will also determine whether you are tonifying or reducing. See the commonly used points above.

How Much Moxa to Use

Moxa sticks	In general, use the stick for 10-15 minutes on each point using something like the Sparrow Pecking method or until the skin starts to turn pink or reddish.

Cones	3-7 cones for each point or until the skin turns pink or reddish. Some patients require, some less. Stimulation intensity is different for each person and disease condition. Stronger, younger people can tolerate more than an older, weaker person. A person with an upper excess combined with a lower xu (such as Liver Yang rising upward with an underlying Liver Yin xu) can take only a little of this heat. Do moxa in the lower part of the body and use fewer and smaller cones so that you are not adding too much heat. If you do it this way you are guiding the heat downward.
Bigger cones and more units applies to:	• Young, strong men • Use in the lower back, lower abdomen, thick skin, and big muscle areas • Use for Yang collapse and/or severe cold syndromes with a long history of disease.
Small cones, less units applies to:	• Women, children, elderly people, weak patients. • Use in the head, chest, four limbs, thin skin, and thin muscle areas. • Use for wind cold damp Bi syndromes, upper excess + lower deficiency syndromes.

CHAPTER 3
Moxibustion Precautions
and Contraindications

Written Consent!

First and foremost: explain what you are going to do, expected sensations, and that there could be small blisters and/or scar formations. *Have patient sign an informed written consent.* Be very clear and make sure they understand!

> *Have the patient sign an informed written consent!*

That's important enough that I needed to say it twice.

Patient Positioning

Position patient suitably. Usually, that is in a lying down position either supine or prone.

You want to be sure your moxa cones are not going to drop onto the table. You want the bottom of your cones, assuming you are using cones, to be flat and parallel with the earth so that the heat of the burning moxa is going up through the top of the cone.

If you are using moxa on the side, put the patient in a side-lying position to use cones on the skin or on cakes, garlic, ginger, etc.

Be sure when you remove the cones that you don't drop or drag them across any other body parts either. That's why I recommend those needle trays above.

Yang Hyperactivity + Yin Xu Heat

This is something like Liver Yang rising and an underlying Yin xu with xu heat as we talked about above. Use caution here because you don't want to add more heat to the situation. Use smaller and fewer cones to help anchor the Yang, but not so much that you increase the already-hot internal situation.

General Precautions

1. Observe your patient's facial reactions during moxibustion and adjust the intensity of the heat in time to avoid causing burns.

2. Patients in a coma, who have numbness of the skin and/or extremities, diabetes patients with neuropathy, local nerve damage, paralysis, etc. will all require extreme care and attention.

3. When using indirect moxibustion, protect your patient's skin from falling ashes. Those hurt like mad and cause patients to jump. Not so good since we are talking pointy objects and fire.

4. I've been taught to check the skin temperature between cones or stick applications with my own fingers to verify. Some patients don't have fantastic sensation, so they might not know. I find that if I use the back of my hand I get a better temperature reading than if I use the pads of my fingers.

5. Apply burn cream to the area when you are done with the moxibustion.

Contraindications

*   Do *not* apply direct or scarring moxa to:
    o   Face
    o   Genitalia
    o   Vicinity of large blood vessels or joints
    o   Pregnant patients in the area of the abdomen or lumbosacral areas.

MANAGEMENT OF BURNS

We're using fire. Sometimes there are burns, hence the written and signed informed consent. As a rule, I send patients home with a little of the miracle Chinese burn cream and tell them how to use it. I always keep a few small containers around the office I can put it into. Doesn't take much at all, just a little blob about the size of a dime.

What happens if moxa leaves a blister? Infection is your primary concern. For moderate or severe burns, refer your patient to the emergency room.

Small blisters will heal on their own, but for larger blisters, puncture them with a sterile needle, drain them, then dress them with sterile gauze.

This page intentionally left blank.

SECTION 2
Three Edged Needle Technique

This is a fancy way to say "bleeding techniques." That might sound pretty medieval in some respects, but we're not talking about using leeches here; we're talking an ancient technique that employs either a three-edged needle or a simple lancet to prick points

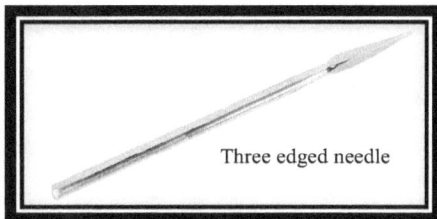

Three edged needle

to remove a few drops of blood in an extremely strategic manner. OK, sometimes it's a little more than a few drops, but never cups or pints!

While looking around for the history of bleeding therapies in China, I came across this terrific site. Take a look and get a good visual idea of some of the principles and methods you will find in this section.

http://www.chinesebloodletting.com/

This page intentionally left blank.

CHAPTER 4
Introduction to
Three Edged Needle Technique

Bloodletting is an old medical modality that was practiced in ancient China, Greece, Egypt, and Europe. Like acupuncture, it probably began with the use of sharp implements to lance and drain infected wounds and bites.

This practice has been strongly disavowed in western medicine due to its' extremely poor applications in the past four hundred years or so. Stories abound about political celebrities who were bled to death by well meaning physicians removing pints and pints of blood in an attempt to cure ailments.

In Chinese medicine, however, the story is quite different. Practiced according to tradition and with appropriate techniques, Chinese bleeding therapies release a few drops of blood to improve the flow of both Qi and Blood to specific areas. This can improve conditions such as accumulations of toxic heat, swellings, pain, Qi and Blood stagnation and stasis, organ and meridian excesses, blocked channels and orificies, migraines, and more.

Three edged needle therapies or bloodletting therapies are indicated for acute conditions, excesses, heat accumulations, localized swelling and numbness, and some pain syndromes.[4]

---

[4] http://www.itmonline.org/arts/bleeding.htm

The area is usually pricked to stimulate bleeding, then gently squeezed to release between 3 and 10 drops of blood. This therapy can be repeated every two to three days, alternating between one side of the body and the other each time.

Bleeding therapies are *not* recommended for anyone who has an excessive bleeding problem (hemophiliacs, people on blood thinners, those who bruise extremely easily, etc.), anemia, low blood pressure, or patients who are pregnant.

MATERIALS NEEDED

In order to use the Chinese bloodletting techniques, you need something that can puncture the skin cleanly and easily and that you can close with nothing more than pressure with a clean cotton ball.

The traditional type of bloodletting needle in Chinese medicine was originally called a lance type needle and looked like a very small version of a spear.

The three-edged needle now is usually made of stainless steel and is around 5-7 centimeters in length. The ones sold in the United States are commonly the disposable type with a three-edged triangular head. The three edges are sharp and easily puncture the skin. In other countries you might find the sterilizable versions. These can puncture more deeply than some of the alternatives.

The other common tool you will see in use in Chinese bloodletting therapies is a simple, disposable lancet like you see in use for testing blood types and testing for blood sugar levels. These work great and are easy to carry in your clinic pack. Their downside is that they do not prick very deeply and you might need something that does.

In addition to either a three-edged needle or lancet, you need some basic cleanup and personal protective equipment (PPE).

Equipment	Brief discussion
Paper towels	Get soft ones. Wiping on skin can be kind of sensitive for some people. Better to give them a pleasant experience. I keep several rolls of this around my office.
Blood spill kit	This was discussed in the first book, *Acupuncture Techniques 101: Safety, CNT, and Needling Techniques*, which is available on Amazon[5] in both digital and print formats.
PPE – personal protective equipment	This was covered in the first book as well. I'd like to specifically mention • Latex or nitrile gloves • Protective eyewear • Clinic coat You have microcuts in your hands most of the time. It would suck to get an infection just because you didn't have gloves. Eyewear is to keep blood from getting in your eyes. The clinic coat protects your clothing and also protects from cross-contamination too.
Cotton balls and an alcohol dispenser	Alcohol acts as a solvent to keep blood from clotting on the surface. This keeps the blood flowing when you are doing bleeding procedures. You need that in some places, especially where there isn't much padding and you are bleeding capillary areas.

[5] Calhoun, Catherine D., L.Ac. *Acupuncture Techniques 101: Safety, CNT, and Needling Techniques*, 2019. Cats TCM Notes Press. ISBN 1070169552.

Bleeding therapy is indicated for conditions of excess, of heat, for blood stagnation, pain, and for acute disorders. Functions, or what a bleeding technique does, include:

Indication/Function	Brief discussion
Clear heat and remove toxins	One application for this might be treating shingles. You can bleed around the edge of the lesions, which releases heat and toxicity in the area and improves s/sx greatly.
Remove blood stagnation	Blood stagnation and the poor blood flow that results to the affected area can display as pain and tightness in an area. As an example, look back to point #2 under the Application heading above. I mentioned that back pain can be linked to distended and/or dark vessels showing around the crease at the back of the knee. Pricking and bleeding those dark vessels can release stuck/stagnant blood and increase blood flow to the local and related areas.
Reduce swelling	This could be swelling from trauma, from a bug bite, or from Blood and Qi stagnation.
Open the channels and stop pain	Blockage/stagnation of blood and blockage/stagnation of Qi both cause pain. Opening the channels will release this stagnation and relieve pain.
Invoke resuscitation	Since bleeding therapies can open the channels and orifices, it can be used to resuscitate people who have the right differentiation/diagnosis for this.

CHAPTER 5
Bleeding Technique Methods

When you are applying bleeding therapies, you are removing a small amount of blood from either a capillary bed or a blood vessel, depending on the vascular structure of the point/s you choose to bleed. In this chapter we will discuss use of the bleeding implements, how to bleed from capillary beds and from blood vessels, and some treatment strategies.

PREP THE POINT

Once you identify the point/s you are going to use, you need to prep them for bleeding. You obviously need to do all the CNT preparation, but you also need to bring the blood to the surface.

If you are bleeding a point in a capillary bed that can include tapping (ok, really gentle slapping), rubbing with a medium vigorousness, squeezing, or light pinching on the point to make the skin pink, signaling the arrival of the blood to the tissue.

You might keep cupping equipment close by also for points on the skin that might not bleed readily (like bleeding at Bladder 17 on the back).

USING BLEEDING EQUIPMENT

How you bleed something depends on where you want to bleed and what implements you are using.

Bleeding with a lancet

This technique is the easier of the two. Why? Because lancets, especially the kind with the removable plastic cap, have a limited penetration distance and are a constant gauge in diameter.

To use these, find your target vessel or point within a capillary bed, put the point of a disposable lancet close to it and pop it, then you bleed it. If the blood stops too soon, swipe the pricked point with a cotton ball moistened with alcohol, which acts as a clotting factor solvent, and bleed it again.

This keeps you from needing to poke more holes in your patient, which they will appreciate because this doesn't exactly feel pleasant.

To finish, use a clean unused cotton ball to press against the pricking point and stop the final bits of blood flow.

Bleeding with a three-edged needle

This takes a little more finesse than using a lancet. Because the point of a three-edged needle flares outward from the tip and because each edge can cut the skin, you need to understand how deep you want the point to penetrate and you need to penetrate the skin cleanly, leaving as little damage as possible.

I use three-edged needles for bleeding vessels and lancets for bleeding points within capillary beds and at the jing well points. Why? 1) You don't need to go very deep for the capillary beds or jing well points, so a lancet works fine and 2) three-edged needles are significantly more expensive than lancets.

To use a three-edged needle well, focus less on the downward stroke that penetrates the skin and more on the upward stroke. This is a *lifting* technique, as if you are trying open an upward exit for the blood and are trying to lift it out of the capillary bed or blood vessel.

Here is how. Again, a written description is no substitute for your professor's advice and guidance. Don't make your instructor send me an e-mail telling me how tired they are of you arguing with them and saying, "Well, it says on CatsTCMNotes…" Listen to your teachers. It's why you've hired them.

Three-edged needle method

1. Locate the point or vessel you want to bleed. Estimate how deeply you need to go to penetrate it. You will get a better bleed from a vessel if you puncture both the front and back of the vessel.

2. Start at an oblique angle with the tip of the three edged needle aimed *very* close to the point you are pricking.

3. Simultaneously strike the target point and lift upward. Focus on the vertical feeling and the sensation of lifting. The strike is actually at the upswing of the vertical lift.

   This is an energetic thing. Do your Qigong exercises from the previous book!

4. Bleed the point.
   If you are pricking a vessel and do it well, the blood should flow easily, but you may have to press and squeeze around the area to bring the blood forward.

   If you are bleeding a specific vessel rather than a capillary bed, always puncture *through* the vessel so you have punctured both sides. This functions as kind of pressure regulator so that the blood keeps flowing as long as you need it to, sort of like when you poke a small hole into a can of liquid you need to empty. What I'm saying is you can't be timid or ginger about this. You have to be decisive and moderately bold and it takes some practice.

You can always use the cotton ball/alcohol trick to keep it flowing if you need to.

5. When you have released enough blood for this procedure, press and hold with a clean unused cotton ball to stop the blood flow.

Learning exercise

Practice this technique *a lot* before you do it on a human!

Level 1
Start with a couple of layers of paper and a ballpoint pen. Practice the strike/lift until you see *only a dot on the paper* rather than a dot and a small line. A small line attached to the dot means you did not have a clean strike/lift.

Level 2
Move on to several layers of paper and a three-edged needle. Mark light X's on the paper. Practice the strike/lift until you see only a dot on the paper in the center of the X with a decent amount of penetration and *no line* cut into the paper by the point of the needle.

Level 3
Now practice with an apple and a three-edged needle. Again, practice the strike/lift and various depths of strike. Be sure you can strike/lift at a variety of depths reliably.

BLEEDING TECHNIQUE APPLICATIONS

There five major types of manipulations or therapy styles you can use when doing bleeding:

1. Spot pricking
   Bloodletting at a single point. As an example, you can prick the top of the ear at the ear apex to treat active migraines. You usually only puncture a single point for spot pricking.

2. Scattering (aka clumping) pricking
   Using this method, you puncture a couple of points in an area. This is often used in combination with cupping to release blood. This is often used for sores, sprains, Bi syndrome, tinea infections, rashes, etc.

3. Blood vessel pricking
   By blood vessel, I mean pricking certain veins on or near an acupuncture point to release stuck or stagnant blood. People with chronic back pain, for instance, will often have dark blood vessels visible at the popliteal crease or popliteal fossa (at the back of the knee). Pricking and bleeding these vessels (the general Bl 39 and Bl 40 areas) can give a very deep release for back pain. Other areas where vessels are pricked are at the cubital crease (PC 3 and Lu 5 area), and the Taiyang area on the temple (can be a great way to treat chronic migraines, fyi).

4. Fibrous tissue broken picking
   This is a way of treating fibroid or scar tissues. We won't cover that much here. There are other ways that are less painful, though this may be suitable for severe cases.

5. Bloodletting and cupping
    I mentioned this one in #2 above. This is also called
    "wet cupping." In this method, covered more thoroughly
    in the cupping section to follow, you use your three-
    edged needle or lancet to prick the skin then place a cup
    over it to encourage bleeding.

COMMONLY USED POINTS FOR BLEEDING THERAPY

There are some points on the body that are routinely used for
bleeding. The table that follows outlines which and for what.

Condition	Points you could bleed for that
Red painful eyes (i.e., conjunctivitis)	Bleed the Taiyang point and the Ear Apex point
Sore throat	Bleed Lung 11 and LI 1 These are jing well points at the distal end of the thumb and index finger respectively, powerful points to release heat in the respiratory system.
Fever	Bleed Ear Apex, Shi Xuan, and the jing well points for fevers.
Sunstroke	Bleed PC 3 and Bl 40 to release heat. Both of those are at the limb creases – the elbow and the back of the knee. These are he sea points and blood flow here is pretty strong. It's a great place to cool the blood pretty quickly. These are points commonly used for excessive heat when little kids spike fevers – a bag of frozen peas at the elbow and knee creases will cool them off pretty quickly. You can use gua sha here too for the same purpose, though bleeding is faster for a case of sunstroke.
Acute lumbar sprain	Bl 40 and any ashi points that are tender.

Condition	Points you could bleed for that
Swollen joints	Bleed local points around the affected joints, especially when joints feel hot/warm to the touch or are swollen from blood stagnation.
Acne	There is a vein on the back of the ear you can bleed to help release heat and toxicity from the face.
Syncope	Fainting, folks. Bleeding at the shi xuan and jing well points will open the channels and assist in resuscitation.
Hypertension	Ear apex. This is a microsystem type of thing. Top of the ear is similar to the top of the body, the head. Bleeding here can lower blood pressure by release stagnation.
Indigestion	Bleed si feng. These are extra points on the palmar side of the hand. You will find these in the center of the proximal inter-phalangeal joints of the fingers.

This page intentionally left blank.

CHAPTER 6
Precautions and Contraindications for Bleeding Therapies

You knew this was coming, right? Blood borne disease transmission possibility increases multiple fold here.

- Use disposable three edged needles, disposable lancets, or be sure you have fantastic sterilization procedures in place if you use re-useable three edged instruments.
- Wear gloves! I recommend you double up here.
- Clean the points after rubbing the area
- Dispose of used needles in a sharps hazardous waste container. If you can squeeze out the paper towels or cotton balls you used to catch the blood and they drip, then they need to go in a hazardous waste bio bag. Check your local regulations for this.
- Wash your hands immediately before and immediately after bleeding techniques are applied.

PATIENT POSITIONING

This is paramount. . . right after the CNT thing. . . Choose the best position that lets the blood flow easily in the affected area, but also keeps your patient safe. Let me give you three examples to illustrate what I'm talking about.

Example 1: Popliteal crease for back pain

The chief complaint is left side back pain. You do your assessment and determine that this is likely a Qi and Blood stagnation problem. You look at the back of the leg and see a dark obvious vessel at Bl 40, so you decide to bleed it. These are a bit deep sometimes, so you decide to use a 3-

edged needle to do the bleeding technique rather than a lancet.

What's the best position for your patient? You could lie them face down, prick it with the 3-edged needle and try to squeeze some blood out, but that's a rookie move. And I ought to know, because I made that rookie move a few times before someone showed me a better way.

First, you want gravity to assist you. Stand that patient up, but you have to do so in a way that is safe. People sometimes faint when they see blood or even when you do bleeding techniques, especially at the back of the knee.

1. Have your patient lean on the acupuncture table on their elbows so that most of their weight is on the table.

2. The leg you are going to bleed rests on the floor with the knee straight.

3. Locate the vessel, use alcohol and a cotton ball to swipe it clean then gather all of your materials.

4. Get a big wad of paper towels ready, prick the vessel and hold the paper towels really close to catch the blood. Sometimes it just oozes out, but sometimes that sucker is under pressure and it will stream a couple of feet. (I lost a good pair of clinic pants to this procedure once because I wasn't quick enough on the draw with the paper towels. It was a dramatic bleeding!) When it does this it is *not* an arterial spurt, but a sustained 'fountain' of what is clearly venous return blood that lasts a few seconds.

Gravity is assisting the blood flow this way and if your patient faints, their weight will fall on the table rather than them falling on the floor.

Example 2: Front of the knee

Same limb, same basic location, but the front of the knee instead of the back of it. There are two Master Tung points on the front of the knee just below the edge of the patella along the margin of the patellar ligament called "Upper Lip and Lower Lip." I use Upper Lip to treat genital herpes and lichen sclerosus and find it works very well with bleeding therapy. To bleed these points I do this:

1. I have the patient sit on the lower edge of the acupuncture table (where the feet usually go) with her knees over the edge and her feet supported on a small step stool and/or pillows so that it's comfortable to be there. I have the patient lean back on her wrists or on her elbows.

    If she faints in this position she's going to fall backwards onto the table rather than onto the floor or forward onto me.

2. I gather my materials and prepare the site I'm going to use (roll up the pants leg, swab the site) and get myself all CNT type prepared.

3. When everything is ready to go, I pinch the skin with medium pressure over and over again to make the area red and get the blood flowing. I then reach over and grab and ear probe and press it firmly against the point I'm going to prick to make an impression which I use as my pricking target.

4. I prick the point and squeeze the tissue around it to make it bleed. I use a cotton ball moistened with

alcohol to swipe over the pricking point when the bleeding slows. I want to get 10+ drops out of the point to really relieve the lesions in the genital area.

Bleeding in this position is comfortable for the patient and gives them a soft place to land should they faint.

Example 3

I once had a friend who had gotten a very bad cold that turned into bronchitis. After the 3rd round of antibiotics and meds and still no relief from the coughing, she asked me for help. I evaluated and saw a giant looking dark, distended blood vessel right around Lung 5 and decided to bleed it. She was already laying face up on the acupuncture table so I had her drop her arm over one edge and supported it in a chair and some stacked pillows, which I had draped with a clinic sheet.

This kept her arm comfortable, kept her in a safe position, and yet still allowed a gravity assist. I could have also used more pillows to prop her upper body at an angle.

I did the bleeding procedure. About a tablespoon's worth (~15ml or so) of very dark thick black colored blood oozed out of the prick point before the blood turned a normal looking color. It was extremely creepy cool. Her cough was gone the following day and her lungs cleared significantly. Her body finished healing about four days later.

There are some instances in which you just don't do bleeding techniques. Nada. Don't.

Proceed with extreme caution	• Weak • Aged • Anemic

Just don't!	• Pregnant patients
	• Anyone susceptible to spontaneous bleeding:
	  ○ Hemophiliacs
	  ○ People on pharmaceutical blood thinners
	  ○ People taking blood moving/anti-blood stasis herbal medicine
	• **Never bleed an artery!**
	You only bleed veins and capillary sized arterial areas such as at the apex of the ear or that Master Tung point on the knee I mentioned earlier.

This page intentionally left blank.

SECTION 3
Cutaneous Needle Therapy

When you insert an acupuncture needle, that is a *sub*cutaneous needle therapy. When you are using *cutaneous* needle therapy this means you are using only the point of a needle to stimulate the surface of the skin.

THE THEORY UNDERLYING CUTANEOUS NEEDLE THERAPY

The *Neijing* says that the collateral channels and vessels of the twelve major meridians supply the cutaneous regions of the body superficially, so occurrence of various disease will start at the skin and sweating pores. Shingles (all of the herpes expressions, really) is a disease that affects the Liver, so it is treated with a formula called *long dan xie gan tang*, which clears Liver fire, cleanses the Liver, and also helps resolve the stagnation of Liver Qi that can contribute to the heat. You can see that this is clearly a Liver thing from a TCM perspective, but what people *notice* about a herpes virus flare is not the liver, but the lesions on the skin. This is a good example of a disease occurrence starting at the skin.

The skin, which is the cutaneous region referred to in the *Neijing*, is closely linked to the jingluo and Zangfu organs, so stimulation in these cutaneous region will activate and regulate the function of both the channels and Yin organs in order to treat diseases. Going back to the shingles example, one of the ways you treat the painful skin lesions and simultaneously clear the Liver fire that is fueling them is to use cutaneous needle therapy around the margins of the lesions. Everything hurts like hell when you have shingles, even a t-shirt touching the skin, so cutaneous needle therapy doesn't feel good when it's happening, but the relief afterwards for a long time is significant.

So to belabor the point, since each of the channels/meridians has it's corresponding domain on the skin and is linked to the organs, this tapping on the skin stimulates not only tissues in the immediate local vicinity, but also the corresponding channels and organs.

CHAPTER 7
Materials for Cutaneous Needle Therapy

Cutaneous needling stimulates the skin without puncturing it deeply. There are several tools you can use to do this kind of stimulation. Probably the oldest method was to hold a few needles at the same time and tap on the skin. You could also do half-insertions and superficial needling and stimulate the cutaneous regions. Honora Wolfe, one of the founders of the Blue Poppy Institute has an interesting video on how to use an acupuncture needle to do this.[6]

CUTANEOUS THERAPY MATERIALS

The most common and convenient way for acupuncturists to do this is to use either a plum blossom needle or a seven star needle.

Seven Star Needle

These are hammer type devices with needles clustered on one end and a flexible handle. You hold the handle as shown in the graphic and

Plum Blossom Needle

Seven Star, Plum Blossom, & proper hold position

apply a tapping stimulation to the skin. The flexibility of the handle gives the hammer head more force and a stronger stimulation on the down-stroke. Note the difference between the seven-star and the plum blossom in the illustration. Also note the different configuration of the type in the proper hold position. These come in a variety of configurations. Choose the type you want for the stimulation you need. Several styles have replaceable

---

[6] https://www.youtube.com/watch?v=gNAU2Y9Fb9Q

heads, which are discarded after use. Some styles are completely discarded.

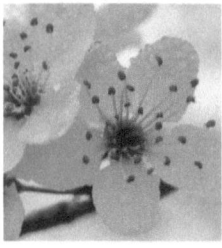 Fun bit of trivia: these types of needles are named after the plum blossom flowers, which have five lobes on the flower. These are traditionally made with five stimulating points. You'll notice on some of the plum blossom needles that there is often a tighter cluster on one side for a stronger and more intense stimulation and for use in very tight areas.

Seven star needles have a greater number of points in a looser cluster. You'd think that would be seven points, but I have one with nine.

FUNCTIONS AND INDICATIONS

Bleeding has five major functions:
- It clears heat and removes toxins from the body.
- Moves stagnant blood and allows for better blood flow.
- Reduces swelling
- Opens the channels to stop pain
- Can be used for resuscitation

For these reasons, bleed therapy can be used to treat excesses, heat in the body, blood stagnation, pain and acute disorders.

CHAPTER 8
Methods of Application

Your instructor will guide you in the proper method of holding and tapping. Then general holding posture looks like the one in the illustration below.

Holding position

This gives you a firm grip, but allows for the flexible handle to apply the best force and spring action.

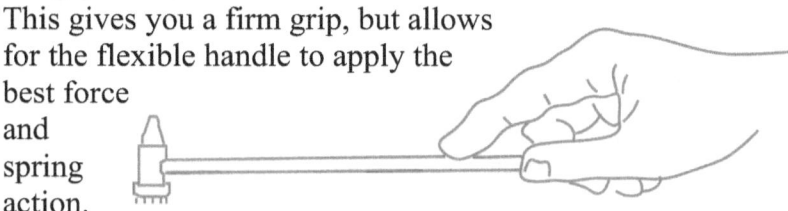

You are going for a bouncing type action and this allows the best bounce.

Tapping Methods

- Tap perpendicularly
  Use the force of your wrist/fingers in a bouncing motion. Tap *perpendicularly* to the surface of the skin to evenly distribute the force.
    - o Hold the head of the instrument so that it strikes at a right angle to the skin, allowing equal force on all of the needle points.
    - o Hold the head 1-2 inches above the surface of the skin.
    - o Tap rapidly flexing only your wrist during tapping (as opposed to your whole arm or forearm – that would give too *much* force).

- Speed of percussion
  Tap at a rate of 70-90 times per minute for approximately 5-10 minutes or until the skin turns pink

  This is the *usual* manner for a medium to mild stimulation. More about stronger stimulations in a moment.

INTENSITY AND VOLUME OF STIMULATION

Now that you know the usual method of stimulation – until the skin turns pink – there are stronger stimulations you can get with cutaneous therapy too.

Stimulation intensity guide

Stimulation	Brief discussion
Mild	Skin turns pink, no bleeding, no pain. Appropriate for: • Elderly, weak, children, pregnant patients Use this level of stimulation for: • Face, head, areas with thin musculature or thin skin tissues.
Moderate	Skin turns red, no bleeding, slight pain. Appropriate for: • Most patients, except very weak ones and very pregnant ones. Use this level of stimulation for: • Anywhere *except* face, head, areas of thin musculature or thin skin tissues. Moderate stimulation is too much, too painful here because there isn't much tissue to pad the nerve endings.

Stimulation	Brief discussion
Strong	Skin turns red, there is some light bleeding, and the procedure is indeed painful. Appropriate for: • Patients with a strong constitution Use this level of stimulation for: • Muscular areas like shoulders, back, low back, buttocks, four limbs

Volume of cutaneous therapy to be applied

This is a judgment call and several factors have to be considered. Do you apply mild, moderate, or strong stimulation? You need to ask yourself several questions to determine this regarding the patient in question.

- What is their body constitution?
  What level of stimulation will their physical condition tolerate? Are they too weak or too sensitive to handle the therapy at all? Are they strong enough to *not* be depleted by this?

- What is this person's age?
  Kids are more sensitive to stimulation due to their high level of Yang, which brings more Qi and more sensation to the skin level. Elderly, very young, and weak patients generally need milder stimulation.

- What is the condition of the disease?
  Is this an acute, chronic, severe, or mild disease presentation? Acute and severe disease might require a more forceful stimulation than a chronic disease.

- What area will cutaneous therapy be applied to? Use the stimulation intensity guide above to help you determine what level of force is applied to a given area.

Area	Brief discussion
Basic tapping and point tapping	This is the most use. It is often used in the back shu areas and can stimulate several points at once. That's really handy for complex conditions, which are pretty common. This method is often used along the Du channel, Bladder channels on the neck, sacrum, and back, on the jiaji points right beside the spinous processes, and on single points anywhere on the body . For single point stimulation many practitioners will use the tight cluster on one end of the plum blossom head.
Tapping along the channel	Great for opening the channel and stimulating the organ that is associated with it. Tap along the channel but only in areas below the knees and elbows.
Tapping in local areas	Tapping in a local area to treat a specific disease manifestation. Examples: • Joint disorders • Skin disorders like numbness, neurodermatitis, rash, tinea, psoriasis, and alopecia. For alopecia, it's probably better to treat right after hair loss starts rather than after long term. In China practitioners also use fresh ginger juice, rubbing it on the skin as well for acute hair loss.

Area	Brief discussion
	The mild damage caused by cutaneous needling here causes an increase in blood flow and stimulates the immune response.
Around the eye, nose, face, and head	Disorders of the eye, with careful mild tapping around the orbital area, respond quite well with cutaneous therapy. Use the cautions about tapping around the face and thin skin areas as discussed already.

DISEASE TREATMENT WITH CUTANEOUS NEEDLE THERAPY

Disease	Area to tap	Intensity
Skin numbness	Affected area	Moderate to strong
Psoriasis	Affected area	Moderate to strong
Alopecia	Affected area Back shu points	Moderate
Acute lumbar sprain	Jiaji points Ashi points + cupping	Strong
Frozen shoulder	Jiaji points Ashi points + cupping	Moderate to strong
Asthma	Jiaji points Lung points Chest	Moderate
Insomnia	Head and neck Jiaji points Yintang and Taiyang Du 20	Mild to moderate
Stomach ache	Back shu points Upper abdomen Stomach channel	Moderate
Abdominal pain	Back shu points Upper abdomen Stomach channel	Moderate
Impotence, dysmenorrhea	Lower abdomen Lower back Sacrum 3 Foot Yin channels	Moderate

This page intentionally left blank.

Chapter 9
CNT, Precautions, Contraindications

There are varying levels of stimulation of the skin in cutaneous needle therapy. Many of them are milder stimulations and you are going for nothing beyond a pinking up of the skin. You might be tempted to skimp on the CNT procedures here, but you can't. Even if you are barely penetrating the skin, you still need to be aware of the risk of infection and cross-contaminations.

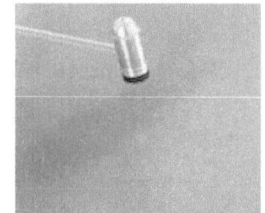

Examine the equipment

- The package containing the whole disposable hammer or the disposable hammerhead should be intact, free of punctures or cuts, and should be clean.

  Re-useable plum blossom and seven star needles are more common in some areas, so if you are using these, be sure to check the head after each sterilization and before each use. Autoclaving can cause a lot of wear and degradation over time. Look for any damaged or hooked points on the head. Discard these and get new ones if you see that. These won't give you the stimulation you want and will cause unnecessary pain and skin tearing.

- The tips of the needles should be level with each other, not "hooked."

- The head and the handle of needle should be firmly joined to avoid possible movement of the head during tapping.

Keep it sterile

Disposable cutaneous needle devices

- Disposable and plastic equipment that cannot be sterilized only on one patient.

- If you are moving from one area of the body to another – i.e. from one limb to another, or from the trunk to the face, the foot to the face, etc. – change devices or change the head on the device. You can definitely cross contaminate between one area and another and cause autogenous infections if you don't.

  Example: one instructor relayed a tale about tinea on the foot being transferred to the face because a practitioner didn't change hammer heads when moving from the Gallbladder channel on the foot to the Gallbladder channel on the face.

  This is why you shouldn't share razors with another person or shave your legs with a razor your husband uses on his face. . . . or let your wife use your razor on her legs. You get the idea.

Re-usable and sterilizable cutaneous devices

Sterilize the cutaneous stimulation devices after each use following standard sterilizing procedures. Always examine the stimulation heads after each sterilization procedure.

Contraindications for cutaneous therapies

Do not use on open wounds, ulcers, or scars. OK, really you can use them around keloid scars, but it will only reduce the nature of the scar, won't resolve it. And you *can* use the technique around the edge of lesions, but not directly on them.

If you do find you are treating a lot of scar tissue, check out Kiiko Matsumo's Japanese style of needling. She gets great results with scar tissues and so do her students. This is a more advanced technique though. Learn this for now and tuck that little bit of info into your "pocket" for later.

Considerations and tips for cutaneous therapy

- The usual sequence of taping is to move from above to below, lateral to medial, Yang to Yin areas.

- When you are stimulating a meridian pathway, a single tap is given every centimeter or so along the pathway. Eight to sixteen taps is generally sufficient to stimulate the meridian.

- Treatments can be given daily, on alternating days, or weekly

- Ten to fifteen treatments over a period of two to three weeks is a common frequency to see for treatment of most chronic diseases.

This page intentionally left blank.

SECTION 4
Gua Sha Therapy

When I was learning gua sha therapy a new professor who had just moved to the United States from China asked me what I was learning in my acupuncture techniques class. When I replied "gua sha," his immediate response was, "Why?! My grandmother knows haw to do that!" He was floored that people in the US do not grow up with this as a common practice.

Gua sha is a common practice in a lot of cultures and is a folk medicine practiced in China by many people, most of whom are not medically trained. It is often used for the common cold, wind cold and wind heat invasions, and for the beginning stages of febrile diseases.

This page intentionally left blank.

CHAPTER 10
Introduction to Gua Sha

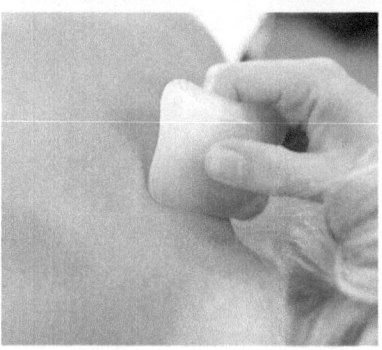

Gua sha is a natural alternative therapy that involves scraping the skin with a smooth edged massage tool, gua sha tool, or other implement to move stagnant Blood, open the channels, eliminate toxins, clear heat, remove early stage pathogenic invasions, and regulate internal organ and channel function by stimulating the cutaneous areas of the body.

When you perform gua sha you use oil on the skin to be scraped, which makes a smoother gua sha stroke and protects the surface of the skin. You scrape until the skin gets red or you begin to see sha spots appearing. You can see them in the photograph just below this heading directly right and below the gua sha tool.

Please note that the gua sha modality is used for relatively mild problems. The term "sha" in gua sha can refer to the spots left behind when you perform gua sha.

It is, however, the same word that is used for something called "sha syndrome," a disease that refers to an invasion of a febrile disease pathogen that then blocks the channels and causes red spots called "sha." The cause of sha syndrome starts with a wind, cold, damp, heat or summer heat invasion and/or an epidemic pathogen which then blocks the channels. S/sx include distended feelings in the chest, head, and abdomen, headaches, pain all over, and feelings of distention and pain in the limbs. If allows to progress, this will show red rashy prickles – sha spots.

If you look back at the second Diagnostics book,[7] the diagnostic theory of the Four Levels describes sha spots that appear in the Ying stage of a warm injured disease where heat in the body is starting to affect the blood. These red rash looking bumps are also referred to as "sha."

Why am I telling you this?

Because if you see a patient who already *has* these red spots, it's too late for gua sha. The disease is already presenting with sha spots, so creating them with a gua sha tool will not release the disease at that stage.

If, however, you see a patient in the early stages of a wind heat, wind cold, or wind damp invasion, you can probably help them out an awful lot if you do gua sha for them in the appropriate areas.

GUA SHA TOOLS

The basic tools for gua sha include a human body, an oil to lubricate and protect the skin, something to scrape with (called a gua sha plate), and paper towels to clean up with.

Commercial gua sha tools can range from fairly expensive jade and rose quartz gua sha plates to way less expensive resin sets. Tools come in a wide array of designs that accommodate different parts of the body.

I bought commercial gua sha tools and special gua sha oil when I was in school, but now my favorite gua sha tools include a ceramic Chinese soup spoon ($1.59 at a local Chinese market in

---

[7] Calhoun, Catherine D. L.Ac. *Diagnostic Skills in Chinese Medicine Book 2: Symptom Analysis and Syndrome Differentiation*, 2019. Cats TCM Notes Press. ISBN: 1097891062.

Austin, but $2.25 on LhasaOMS), a US quarter ($0.25…duh), and organic sesame oil ($7.99 at Whole Foods). I honestly prefer these to any of the special bone and jade tools I bought in school (which now are only on display in my office). However, if I did facial/beauty treatments I would probably take the jade gua sha plate off of the shelf and actually use it.

Tool	Reason for use
Gua sha plate	Different configurations to these and come in several types of materials. There is one that looks like a comb that can be used for scalp stimulation. That helps regulate brain function and increases your intelligence. Another has a wide divot for use along the fingers. Some have curves that can wrap around the bones of the spine . Some look like chisels with softer edges that are used in a variety of ways. You will find some that also have soft points that are used for acupressure stimulation.
Buffalo horn	You can use this tool to scrape over tightness at the back of the neck. The pointed side of the horn is used for acupressure. The horn itself is used as an herbal medicine that clears heat, removes toxins and cools the blood. It does this internally, but also carries those qualities to a gua sha treatment when you use this horn as a scraping tool.
Jade	Jade gua sha tools are cooler than other stones and will help clear heat from the body. Some massage tools as well as many of the facial gua sha tools are made from jade for this reason. This generally requires a very light touch gua sha technique that doesn't raise sha spots.

Tool	Reason for use
	This technique, when applied to the face, also moves Qi and Blood and is part of Chinese beauty culture.
Rose Quartz	Rose quartz gua sha tools are also used on the face and are said to increase skin elasticity and reduce the appearance of fine lines. Egyptian and Greek cultures traditionally used rose quartz to retain youth and beauty. That could be the reason these are showing up on the gua sha scene now.

What about oils?

There are a kabillion choices for oils you could use for gua sha…. But start thinking about the medicinal properties of the ingredients of the oils and whether those properties support what you are trying to accomplish with gua sha in the first place.

Are you trying to help clear a wind heat invasion? Maybe think about using sesame oil as your lubricant of choice for this treatment because it is clear heat well. Is there a ton of muscular tension you are trying to clear by moving Qi and Blood? Then think about something like Tiger Balm or White Flower Oil that has warming and opening qualities to it.

Peanut oil is thick and neutral in temperature. It can improve digestion and holds up well to the scraping motions while protecting the skin, *but* many people are allergic to peanuts, so this isn't the best choice when you don't know for sure about allergies.

Almond oil is another traditional oil used for gua sha. It is neutral in temperature, tonifies Qi and the Jing, and has a phlegm resolving action. This could be a good choice for exterior invasions that result in phlegm build up.

Could you mix some essential oils into your carrier oil (fractionated or organic regular coconut oil, almond oil, etc.)? Absolutely, you can. Look into Snow Lotus oils[8] if this interests you. These are good quality oils formulated from a Chinese medicine perspective.

WHAT GUA SHA TREATS – INDICATIONS

My dad's favorite phrase was "right tool for the job." As you learn the modalities of treatment that we use in Chinese medicine you will learn what works best to treat various disease states. This is what gua sha works well for.

FYI, this is a very terse guide. If you want to know more about gua sha than you are getting here, check out Ayra Nielsen's fantastic book on gua sha.[9]

Indication	Brief discussion
Disease of external origin	• Common cold • Cough • Asthma • Stomach flu • Sunstroke and external heat excesses
Pain	Very effective for musculo-skeletal and abdominal pain. Needling, moxibustion, cupping, and gua sha are actually all quite effective for these things. Sometimes what you choose depends on your patient. I have a heavily tattoo'd patient who is scared silly about needles. He's got a lot of shoulder and neck pain because of his job. (Would you

---

[8] http://www.snowlotus.org/
[9] Nielsen, Arya. *Gua Sha: A traditional technique for modern practice.* Churchill Livingstone Press. ISBN 044305282X.

Indication	Brief discussion
	believe tattoo artist? Not even kidding.) For him I use cupping and gua sha and he gets great relief. Sometimes this choice is a matter of convenience. I've treated the lower back with needles and simultaneously treated the upper back and shoulders with gua sha. You'll figure out what works for you. But I will point out that before you get your acupuncture license you *can't* legally needle (in the U.S. at least), but you *can* do cupping and gua sha to help people get pain relief. I'm just sayin'.
Digestive issues	The digestive tract is connected to the external body via the Wei qi. In newer Chinese medical theories and with newer research, it has been suggested that all of the tissues that have squamous cells – including skin and digestive tract – are related and connected through this association as well. So once again, digestive tract can be affected by treating the skin. This means you can use gua sha to treat acute gastroenteritis as well as dysentery and other damp heat invasions in the digestive tract. You can even treat chronic problems such as Crohn's disease (which manifests with alternating diarrhea and constipation and inflammation in the tract) with gua sha. You can scrape over the affected areas also, both on the front and the back of the body.
Health preservation	This is a light stimulation and uses no oil. Stimulate the Jiaji and both Bladder lines on the back for health preservation.

Indication	Brief discussion
Headaches, insomnia, and poor memory	Stimulate the head and neck.
Sinus problems and allergies	Whether chronic or acute, you can stimulate either side of the nose as well as the upper back – Bladder 12 and 13 areas. Also stimulate the Ren channel and the thymus to help with chronic allergies.
Ringing in the ears	Scape on the side of the ear for this
Blood circulation	Improve blood circulation by scraping in the affected areas.
Chest tightness	Scrape down the sternum, out along the intercostal spaces from the margin of the sternum laterally.

This page intentionally left blank.

CHAPTER 11
Gua Sha Methods

Now that you have selected your tools and your oils (which is probably whatever you instructor has told you to get – and that's a good plan at this stage), you need to know how to use them. There are three basic methods.

Method	Brief discussion
Scraping	• Direct scraping This is what we've been talking about all along – oil on the body, gua sha tool to scrape the surface. In the next chapter we are going to talk about "sliding cupping" which is another form of gua sha. • Indirect scraping This is not commonly used. It's mostly used on kids and very old people who have tender skin or injures easily. Apply a layer of silk or other cloth rather than oil on top of skin, then scrape. Similar to some of the tuina massage techniques.
Drawing method	This is a method of gua sha that uses your fingers rather than a tool. This is mostly used when a pathogen is superficial (at the Wei level). You *pinch* or draw the skin repeatedly until a purple spot appears when you are using the drawing method. This can be used on the neck and head like at the Taiyang, Yintang, and Gb 20 points, and also on the limbs at the cubital and popliteal fossa. For high fevers and mild sunstroke you can use

Method	Brief discussion
	the drawing method around PC 3 or LI 11, and Bl 40.
Bloodletting method	I'm sorry, I don't actually have a lot of data on this. I know you use it when sha spots may already be visible, indicating that the pathogen is deeper - at the Qi or Ying levels in the Four Levels theory.

Gua sha is commonly used on the head, neck, back, chest and four limbs. The method you use for a gua sha stroke is even pressure across the entire length of the stroke. You drag the edge of the tool across the skin rather than

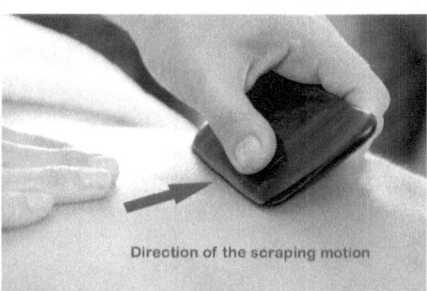

Direction of the scraping motion

pushing it. Place the tool's edge at an oblique angle to the skin and make the length of the stroke with even pressure all the way from the beginning to the end of the stroke.

You repeat this in *one area at a time* until you get the desired effect you want on the skin – pinkness, sha spots, etc. At that point you can then move to another area.

Scrape until you hear a light rasping indicating you are running low on skin lubricant. When you hear that, stop and move the oil around on the body to re-lubricate the area. Try another stroke and make sure you don't hear the rasping. If you do, apply a little more oil.

Be aware of the underlying bone structures. For the most part, you want to slide the gua sha tool along the natural curves of the body between the bones rather than bumping over the top of them like a bunch of speed bumps.

Let's look at what areas gua sha is commonly used and how your move the gua sha tool through this area.

Note that scraping is *not bidirectional!* You only scrape in the direction indicated below.

Area	Brief discussion	Direction/method notes
Head and back of neck	Yintang	Use drawing method here.
	Taiyang	Use drawing method here.
	Gb 20 and back of neck Great for tension headaches	Scrape downwards from Gb 20 parallel to the cervical spine. Go only as far down as the curve of the neck. Repeat these strokes until you see sha spots. You can combine gua sha with acupressure at Gb 20.
Neck	Side of the neck – scalenes	Scrape downwards only. You might have to use your fingers to stabilize the skin. Releases tension in the scalenes. Make your patient aware of the bruising that will occur!
	Gb 20 to Gb 21	Follow the curve of the neck from the Gb 20 point to the Gb 21 point at the apex of the shoulder muscles.
	Neck, shoulders, upper back	Great for exterior invasions, asthma, respiratory problems, pneumonia and more. Scrape downward on the neck and laterally on the shoulders, following the grain of the muscle underneath. Scrape only out to the medial margin of the scapula.
Back	Du channel along the spine	Scrape the spots *between the spinous processes* rather than long stokes across the bony protrusions. Caveat: some practitioners scrape lightly down the Du channel over the

Area	Brief discussion	Direction/method notes
		spinal protrusions, then continue to the 1st bladder channel lines and repeat, completing one line at a time before moving on.
	Jiaji points	These are points ½ cun from the center line of the spine. On these you can stroke *down* the length of the line. I use a corner of a gua sha plate or my trusty Chinese ceramic spoon.
	Bladder channel lines	There are two bladder lines – the first is 1.5 cun from the centerline of the spine, the 2nd is 3 cun from the centerline of the spine. On both of these you can stroke down the length of these channel lines. Same deal – use the corner of the gua sha plate, the short side of it, or something like a Chinese ceramic spoon. You can make your strokes downward in a line. Alternately, you can stroke from the center to the lateral aspect (either from the jiaji points out to the 1st or 2nd Bladder line), following the intercostal spaces between the ribs.
	Lumbar area	Down and laterally are both good motions for this area.
Chest	Great for coughs.	The area you use is between the clavicle bones and above the breasts. If you are scraping in the area of the sternum, the strokes are downward. If you are scraping lateral to the sternum, follow the intercostal spaces and scrape between them starting at the edge of the sternum and scraping laterally along the spaces.

Area	Brief discussion	Direction/method notes
Four limbs	Sciatica area pain	Scrape downward along the grain of the muscle on the buttocks and lower back, also along the affected aspect of the lower leg. That could be along the Gallbladder and/or Bladder channel, sometimes along the Stomach channel on the anterior leg. Always follow the direction of the channel – downward.
	Arm pain, shoulder tightness	On the upper back as described above. *Down* the upper arm along the affected channel.

READING THE SHA SPOTS

You'll notice that sometimes the spots are slow to show and are small even if you are scraping a lot. And sometimes the spots show up quickly and are darker than you expected. What does that mean? What does the color difference mean? What if there are no spots?!

Presentation	What that means
Bright red spots	• Exterior syndrome • Acute disease or short history • Mild case • Good prognosis
Dark red spots and/or purple patches	• Interior disease • Chronic history • More severe, deeper case • Prognosis isn't nearly as good
No sha spots	• Huh! No sha syndrome, no external invasion. • Treatment with gua sha isn't specifically needed, but is good for health preservation.

You can use this same chart as a guide for reading cupping marks. More on that in following chapters.

After Care

Gua sha opens the body to expel pathogens, to move Qi and blood, and to open the channels. It's important to give the body a chance to heal. Make sure your patient knows to :

- Take it easy. No heavy labor. Rest the day of treatment.
- Drink warm water to keep the stomach protected.
- Do not take a cold shower. You don't want the cold invading the body.
- Keep the spots that were treated covered for 24 hours.

1. I make double sure I have a signed written consent form from this patient and that they know they are about to have some hellacious looking bruises. Make triple sure this patient isn't going to be wearing a strapless gown or going on a honeymoon or anything where explaining these marks is going to be problematic!

2. Get my tools together – oil, scraping tools, paper towels for clean up.

3. Position the patient in the best manner for the area I need to treat.

4. Apply oil to the target area, then clean my hands with paper towels as well as possible so the gua sha plates don't go shooting across the room!

5. Treat with gua sha using medium firm strokes with even pressure that drag the edge of the gua sha tool at an oblique to 30° angle.

   Keep treating in one area until you get the level of sha spots you feel is appropriate for the condition and patient.

   You will note that your applied oil starts to stack up as you scrape the skin. You'll hear your gua sha tool make a rasping sound on the skin when you need to apply more oil. Try redistributing the oil that's stacked up instead of applying more. It makes clean up (step 7) a whole lot easier. Use you hand to redistribute the oil and keep scraping. Do this each time you hear the rasping. If you have to apply more oil, do it in very small amounts or you'll be cleaning that stuff up forever.

6. Move to the next area and repeat until the whole area you have chosen to influence has been treated.

7. Gently *blot* the oil off of your patient with paper towels rather than wiping the oil off. The skin will tender and they might have a lot of pain if you wipe. I also recommend buying the softest paper towels you can find. Viva has a variety that feels more like cloth than paper. That's always done well.

   You need to get as much oil off as possible. Leaving enough oil on someone to stain their clothes makes them angry enough to never come back. Oil stains are hard to get out in the laundry. Be thoughtful about this.

CHAPTER 12
Precautions and Contraindications

PRECAUTIONS AND TIPS FOR TREATMENT

Tip	Brief discussion
Patient position	Position patient so muscles are not too tight and not too loose. Example: To gua sha the neck, look for neck folds when the patient is lying face down. Very muscular people, people with loose skin, and overweight people will have folds that are hard to gua sha around. Have these folks either sit up and treat this way, or angle the face cradle far enough down so that the rolls and wrinkles disappear.
Clean the gua sha tools	There is no need to sterilize, but you do need to clean your gua sha tools with soap and water and then wipe them with alcohol to disinfect.
Always apply guasha oil	Unless you are doing a health maintenance treatment. Listen for the rasping sound that means you are running out of oil in that area.
Angle, direction of scrape	Angle at which you scrape should always be oblique to the plane of the skin so that you don't cut it. Never hold the gua sha plate or tool perpendicular to the skin. Always drag the edge of the tool rather than pushing it to avoid cutting the skin.
Strength of stroke	Strength of your stroke should be even from beginning to end of stroke.
Direction of stroke	Direction of stroke is *always* one way – never drag the tool back and forth!!

Tip	Brief discussion
When to move	Finish one area completely before moving to another area of stimulation. Get the sha spots before you move on.
Stimulation intensity	Stroke until sha spots appear completely. Use light stimulation for the first treatment, for aged patients, weak patients. Go for a pink/red to the skin only. You also use this kind of stimulation for a health maintenance treatment.
After treatment	Have the patient rest, drink warm water, avoid cold showers for 24 hours, don't swim in cold water for 24 hours, and keep the area covered for 24 hours.
Frequency of treatment	Can repeat every 3-7 days after sha spots appear.

CONTRAINDICATIONS

Never use gua sha for:

- Patients with bleeding problems
  Hemophilia, easy to bruise, patients on high doses of blood thinners, people who hemorrhage easily, people who get purpura easily, people with leukemia.

- Those who have open wounds, masses, scars, or infections in the area you plan to treat.

- Do not gua sha in bony areas.

- Pregnant patients: do not use on the lower back or abdomen. Avoid the 'contraindicated during pregnancy' points like Gb 21.

SECTION 5
Cupping Therapy

I bet most of us have practiced cupping even before we learned what it was. Don't believe me? Most of us have sucked the air out of the inside of a cup so that it stuck to our faces. That, in a nutshell, is cupping.

The way we are going to do it is a little different, but the effect is the same. Stay tuned and learn about basic fire cupping with glass cups, therapeutic methods, and why the hell Kylie Jenner did that weird thing with her lips a couple of years ago.

This page intentionally left blank.

CHAPTER 13
Introduction to Cupping

Cupping is a container of some kind to which you apply negative pressure to create a suction in the container. People figured this out all over the world a *long* time ago. There is an Egyptian papyrus[10] written around 3500 years in the past that details cupping. There's an Arabic word – "hijama" – cupping![11] Hippocrates, Galen, and Herodotus, famous Greek physicians used it and wrote about it too. When I was a kid my neighbor, Mrs. Gamez, heard me coughing and wheezing and got permission from my mom to do a procedure I now know as cupping. She had learned it from her great grandmother. Ge Hong, a physician in the Jin Dynasty who lived about 2000 years ago, popularized a saying, "Acupuncture and cupping, more than half of the ills cured."

See what I'm saying? Cupping has a long and worldwide history. It's been proven effective (even if Wikipedia has a strong anti-alternative medicine bias and says it's crap). We all know it, we've all used it for hundreds of generations. It was originally called the "horn method" because hollow animal horns were used for the cup part. Later bamboo cups were introduced as part of cupping therapy.

Horns and cups are still used – obviously, because there aren't a whole lot of photographs floating around from 3000 years ago. As you can see from the graphic below, fire is used with bamboo, horn, and glass cups to burn out the oxygen. This creates a negative pressure, which in turn creates the suction effect.

---

[10] https://www.ncbi.nlm.nih.gov/pubmed/15586450
[11] https://www.ncbi.nlm.nih.gov/pubmed/28494847

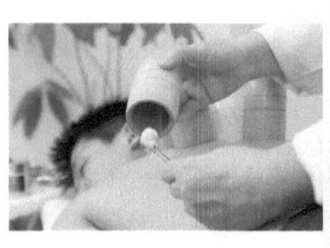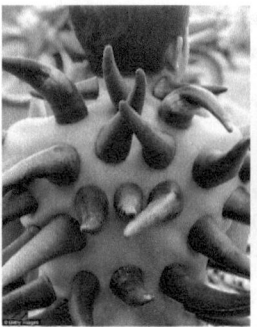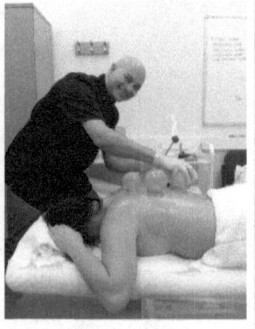

Cupping with bamboo, horn, and glass cups.
And do those horns look like something off Agents of S.H.I.E.L.D. or what?

The important thing, regardless of whether you use bamboo, horn, glass, porcelain, silicone, baby food jars, or pneumatic cups, is the negative pressure. That's what has the medicinal effect: the action and the application of cupping.

MATERIALS YOU WILL NEED

Though there is a wide array of cupping materials you could use, start with **standard glass cups**. They have a number of benefits, especially if you are just learning all of this.

Benefits of heavy glass cups

Benefit	Brief discussion
Cost effective	At the time of this printing, you can purchase a 3 cup starter pack for less than $10. You can buy individual cups in various sizes to expand your set, getting the sizes you use most, for $3-5 USD per cup.
Durable	I'm actually kind of amazed at how durable glass cups are. I carried 12 of them around daily for many years and never even chipped one. And I'm not exactly careful either. My dad, in a moment of frustration when I was in high school, once declared that I could tear up a steel ball with a rubber hammer, so the fact that I still use the glass cups I collected when I started school in

Benefit	Brief discussion
	2007 is a testament to their fortitude!
Sterilizable	But you *can* wash them, run them through a double sterilization process, and you have reliably clean cups that aren't going to cross-contaminate. Since they are glass they are resistant to bleach, which you can't say about the pneumatic cupping sets or the suction cup sets. The small soft parts in those will break down over time after repeat bleach soaks. Remember that some nasty viruses can live up to a week on a sterile surface. The ability to sterilize these should not be discounted! If you're doing a combination of cupping and bleeding, there's absolutely no way anything other than a solid glass cup is going to ever be completely free of tissue and blood particles (despite what you will routinely see in videos and internet articles). You could argue that the silicone cups could be used this way and you *can* put them through an autoclave, but silicone has tiny pores in the material. I don't trust it. And you can't get the level of suction in a silicone cup that you can in glass. Some sets of glass cups are autoclave safe, but many are not. Check with the manufacturer of yours to find out.
Fire cupping	If you think fire *spinning* is cool, watch people's eyes go wide when you break out the glass cups, the fire, and start suctioning those things onto a human body! You can't do that with silicone, plastic, or even glass pneumatic cups. OK, you could do it with bamboo cups and horns too, but in a clinical environment glass is easier to clean and sterilize. (If you're going to be providing cupping at a heavy metal event or a Renaissance faire

Benefit	Brief discussion
	however, definitely go with the horns. And wear a Viking helmet when you do. And send me a photo!)
Smooth edges	Glass cups have a nice wide, smooth edge for sliding cupping. The cup shape gives you a great grip for this and the lip won't cut the skin when you slide it around. The set pictured here also has finger grips on the larger cups so you can slide more easily. You can do this with *some* pneumatic sets, but many of those hare sharper edged, especially the plastic sets. Always check the edges of your cups for burs, nicks, chips, etc. before use for both sliding and static cupping. (Static cupping means applying a cup and leaving it in place. Sliding cupping means applying oil to the target area, then applying the cup and sliding it around the area in a type of gua sha/massage combo.)
They feel good	They just feel good on the skin when they are applied. If it's wintertime you can run the flame around the lip for a moment to warm it, which makes it feel more comfortable when you apply it. They also feel better when you remove them than the thinner edges of other types of cups because of that thicker lip around the opening.

Benefit	Brief discussion
Needling and cupping	There is a method of cupping in which you insert a needle and then apply a cup over it. It's far easier to do that with glass cups than with any other kind.

Other materials you are going to need

In addition to cups (duh), you need some other stuff too.

The most common method of cupping is often referred to in Chinese medical literature with the rather charming sounding name of "fire twinkling method." There are two other methods called fire throwing and cotton attaching methods. All of these require a similar set of materials.

In addition to a set of glass cups, you are going to need:

Items needed	Brief discussion
Cotton balls	You will soak these in alcohol and light them as your fire source. I recommend getting the organic cotton variety instead of the cheaper versions. Most "cotton balls" aren't cotton at all, but are made from cheaper, bleached synthetic fibers like nylon and polyester. As of this printing, organic cotton balls are about $4 for a pack of 80 while the cheap ones are $3 for 200. I know that sounds like a big difference, but do you really want to breathe burning toxic fumes by lighting cheap cotton balls on fire? No. Not exactly the healing environment you are trying to create. If cost is really a concern, get true cotton for fire cupping and use the less expensive ones for day-to-day use like swabbing points and pressing to stop bleeding.

Items needed	Brief discussion
Long pair of lockable, stainless steel forceps	You will use these to hold the cotton ball and light it. Make sure they are long enough to keep you from getting burned, but short enough that you can use them effectively. Locking forceps The "lockable" variety will make holding a burning cotton ball a lot easier. You will already have enough to think about without worrying about dropping a burning ball of fire.
95-91% isopropyl alcohol	This is the fuel for the fire. 95% is the standard concentration in some locations. 91% is common in the U.S.
Alcohol pump	You probably already have one. Be sure you have one that is stable and easy to use. Some of the portable ones require a fairly hard press and that's much more difficult to manage than the non-portable kind. I like this version→. Even if you have to carry it around empty and put a little alcohol in it for cupping purposes, you'll thank me for this later.
Jar with a lid	You can use this much like you did for moxibustion. Drop your used, ashy cotton balls into this jar to extinguish them safely and know that nothing is smoldering.
Moxa stick snuffer or needle tray	The stuff you use for moxibustion will work great (See Section 1). The snuffer is a nice place to rest the forceps holding your cotton ball in between cup applications.
Candle or lighter	I recommend the candle. Much easier to light an alcohol soaked cotton ball and hold

Items needed	Brief discussion
	the cup in the other hand this way.
Burn cream	Just in case. . .

ACTIONS AND APPLICATION OF CUPPING

Cups are applied at strategic locations on the body to create a therapeutic effect.

Action	Discussion
Moves Qi and Blood	This has a pain relief effect for areas of tightness and pain that have their root in stuck or stagnant Qi and blood. Used in local areas of stagnation either as a static cup or in sliding cupping.
Expels wind and cold	And thus good for treating wind cold /damp/phlegm, etc. Often used in the upper back – Bladder 11-15 area and outward laterally. Sliding or static cupping. (I've used it to pull out heat too – Du 14 is a nice place to put a cup to help the body cool down.)
Dissipates	Dissipates swelling and clumping, clears toxic heat. Can remove toxins if you couple it with a bleeding therapy. Used in local areas of swelling and toxic heat.
Regulates Qi and Blood, stimulates points	Kinda says it all there, doesn't it? Often used at the back shu points for this reason. Good health maintenance treatment. This is often done as a static cupping technique.
Pain	Musculoskeletal pain such as low back pain, stiff neck, shoulder pain, sprains. But also effective for stomach ache, abdominal pain, and dysmenorrhea. You could use cups on front mu, back shu points,

Action	Discussion
	and/or jiaji points. Use mid-back where the back shu for the Spleen and Stomach are for stomach ache, over the Kidney and Bladder back shu for dysmenorrhea.
Wind/cold/damp problems	Wind cold damp can cause bi syndrome that is worse in cold and wet weather conditions, common cold, cough, and asthma. "Bi" means pain in Chinese and usually refers to arthritis, but could by any pain syndrome. Use locally for pain, but you can also use acupuncture points along the path of the channel where the pain is. Take sciatica for instance. Gb 20 is often reactive to palpation when a patient has sciatic pain. I might put a cup on that point then needle or cup other tender or strategic points along the channel. For common cold/asthma/cough, cup the back of neck, upper back. Use smaller cups to concentrate the negative pressure in the cup at Bl 13, Bl 12, Gb 21* (especially for coughing) and Bl 17. You can actually cover the upper back with cups. I've seen it done many a time. Works great. You can also do sliding cupping along the 1st Bladder channel line between Gb 21 and Bl 13/14 You can cup at Lung 1 and Lung 2 if there is enough muscle here. *Remember Gb 21 is contraindicated for pregnant women. Gua sha on the sternum for a cough when you want to descend the rebellious Lung Qi perhaps.
Toxic heat	Sores, carbuncles, swellings, acne, sunstroke, and poisonous snake bite. Use a three edged needle to prick the sore or snake bite open, then use strong suction with a glass cup to suck out the ick. Keep it up until the color of the

Action	Discussion
	blood changes to normal. (It might start off mixed with pus or might be very dark.)

The caveat is acne. Don't do this on the acne spot, but on the jiaji points. Palpate these and feel for texture changes. When you feel something different from the other jiaji points, that's considered reactive. Prick to bleed and cup.

Use PC 3, Bl 40, and Du 14 for sunstroke to release heat quickly. You can prick to bleed and cup on top of it in these spots if needed. |
| Other disease | *So* many others. You can use cups at major points, but are probably best at the back shu and front mu points for specific diseases. Which points those are will depend on what the disease condition is. |

This page intentionally left blank.

Chapter 14
Cupping Basics

Whether you are using a single cup or multiple cups, sliding, or static cupping, the basic method of application for glass cups is the same. Suction (negative pressure) is created with the use of fire inside the cup to burn off the oxygen within.

This is a super simple procedure, but you *are* playing with fire! Do this safely so you don't set your clinic coat or your patient on fire! Let's talk about procedures for both static and sliding cupping first.

The big disclaimer

What your instructor tells you to do is how it's done. Learn it. This is a hands-on experience. You cannot learn this from a book. The stuff that is written here is a reference, a prompt for your memory. It's not the freakin' gospel!

BASIC CUP APPLICATION

These are the basics to make a glass cup stick on the human body in a therapeutic manner. This applies to both static cupping and sliding cupping.

1. You need stuff.
   Get your stuff together, lay out all of your cupping materials, and light your candle. Make sure all of your stuff is pretty close to the patient, like on a surface next to them if possible.

2. Prep the location.
   Identify the location you are planning to cup and have the patient remove clothing from that location. If the

patient has long hair, have them tie it back and get it out of the way.

Many practitioners will apply a very light coating of oil on the target points or area. This gives the skin protection and makes cup removal less surprising and uncomfortable.

3. Get your cotton ball ready.
   Pick up a cotton ball with your forceps and lock it down. Soak this cotton ball in 91-95% alcohol, but not too soaked because you don't want it to drip.

4. Get the cup ready.
   a. Pick up a medium to large sized cup in your *non-dominant* hand.
   b. Move your body so that the cup is within a foot of the patient. Hold the cup with the opening horizontal.

5. Light the fire.
   Pick up the forceps/cotton ball in you *dominant* hand. Light the cotton ball in the candle flame. Put the flame inside the cup and move it around in a circle to burn off the oxygen.

6. Cup to body.
   Move the fire out of the cup and hold it away from the patient. At the same time, immediately apply the cup to the desired location.

Problem solving wimpy suction

If your cups aren't suctioning on well, it's likely one of two reasons:

```
╔══════════════════════════════════════════╗
║                                            ║
║           The bigger the fire,             ║
║         The stronger the suction           ║
║                                            ║
╚══════════════════════════════════════════╝
```

- Your fire is too small.
  Try using a larger cotton ball, which makes a larger flame. Even small cups need a large flame to get good suction.

  Also, make sure you not using 70% alcohol! It often does not burn hot enough. That's why we use 91 or 95% alcohol.

- You are not getting the cup down quickly enough. Keep practicing. Get the cup down quickly, but gently. You need to be physically close to the patient. Hold the cup no more than 12 inches (about 30 cm) above the area to be cupped.

  This is one reason I make sure the patient's clothing is nowhere near where I'm working. I don't have to worry about setting clothing on fire this way!

Some other reasons cups don't stick well or come off on their own:

- Body hair
  When you are cupping hairy people or are cupping in an area with more body hair (like around the base of the skull), you might find that cups don't stick for very long. Hair will weaken the seal around the mouth of the cup and let air leak in. To "fix" this, apply a layer of oil or a balm (like Tiger Balm) in the area, which will give you a better seal.

  If you are treating a *really* hirsute individual, you

might need even more oil.

- Skin folds
  If you are cupping in an area with skin folds or creases, this can also compromise the seal around the lip of the cup. This happens most in my experience on the back near the crease where the arm meets the shoulder. Reposition the cup a little so that it's not on the crease.

- Dry skin
  If you are applying weak cupping (see Chapter 15), you will find that the suction releases faster than you'd like when a person has very dry skin. To fix this, oil them up better and try again.

WHEN THE CUPS ARE ON

Once the cups are on...

- Cover your patient
  Cover them with a light blanket or sheet after the cups are on. Cupping can lower the blood pressure and make the patient feel chilly. If they don't want it immediately, they probably will.

- Don't leave the room!!!
  Never, never, never, never leave the room when the cups are in place. Watch them like a hawk. Why? Because the skin can go from normally colored to "time to take the cup off" very quickly. If you don't take it off in time, blisters can form under the cup. You don't want that.

- Adjusting the level of suction
  Sometimes the cups go on too strong. This takes some practice, but you can press gently with your thumb on the skin right next to the lip of the cup so release just a

little bit of that suction. What generally happened the first 10 or so times I did this was I released too much negative pressure and totally released the cup, so I had to reapply it.

How long do you leave cups on?

Some of this is a judgment call, but there are some basic rules to frame that judgment call.

- Time
  Retain the cups on the body for between 5 and 15 minutes. Go for the low end of the time scale if you are using large cups with a strong suction.

  No more than 20 minutes.

- Color of the skin
  Watch for the skin to change color. When there is stagnation and pain you will often see the skin take on a reddish and/or purple-ish cast and you will often see sha spots form in the cup, similar to what you would see in gua sha.

  The skin doesn't always change color – if it doesn't, don't leave them on more than 20 minutes!

- If applying weak cupping...
  This method is covered in the following chapter and involves very weak suction. With this method, the cups can stay on as long as 30 minutes. See Chapter 15 for more on this.

HOW TO REMOVE CUPS

Once the skin changes colors, or you decide it's been enough time (i.e. 20 minutes or less), you need to remove the cups.

This is a simple procedure in theory, but there are safety aspects you need to know. After the cups have been in place for just a few moments, they will contain vapor, blood particles, body fluids, and internal pathogenic factors that are unique to that patient. If you are doing wet cupping or bleeding cupping, or are cupping in an area with acne or pustules, this is doubly important.

Here's how you remove the cups safely without exposing yourself to the contents of the cup.

1. Stand next to the patient and place the thumb of your non-dominant hand on the skin right next to the lip of the cup *and on the opposite side from where your face is!*

2. Press down on the skin with your thumb while holding on to the cup with your dominant hand.

    If you have done wet or bleeding cupping you will need to follow all CNT procedures including using disposable gloves. You will also need to hold paper towels in the hand you use for the release in such a way that you can catch anything ejected from the cup.

    But vapor and blood particles and such will build up in the cup, so you always need to release it away you're your face regardless of the cupping method you are using (i.e., bleeding cupping, sliding cupping, etc).

3. Remove the cup *gently*.
    Gently pull the lip upward and peeling it away from the

skin. Don't pull it off forcefully or twist it when you remove it. It can hurt to remove them quickly because of the force of the suction around the rim of the cup and how that interacts with the skin.

4. Place the cup in a container for double sterilization.

This page intentionally left blank.

CHAPTER 15
Five Cupping Methods

Are there more than five cupping methods? Of course. But these are the most common in clinic and the most likely to be tested. If you want to know more, there is a terrific book called *Traditional Chinese Medicine Cupping Therapy* by Ilkay Zihni Chirali[12]. It might be in your school library. It's also available on Amazon in both print and digital formats.

SINGLE VS. MULTIPLE CUPS

Single cup use

You can indeed use one single cup on an acupuncture, motor point, or ashi point. This is for use in disorders involving smaller areas.

As an example, when I study or sit at my computer for long hours I get a tightness just medial to the medial margin of my left scapula. If I ignore it, it blossoms into an unignorable tension headache that can last for days. If I have my partner put a cup on it for 15 minutes, then get up and go do something other than sitting at a computer, I'm good.

Here's another example. Let's say you have a patient who comes in with signs and symptoms (s/sx) that point to an early stage wind heat invasion. A single cup to the Du 14 point might be enough to expel it.

---

[12] Chirali, Ilkay Zihni. *Traditional Chinese Medicine Cupping Therapy*. Churchill Livingstone Press. ISBN: B0148JSNYI.

Using multiple cups

The more common thing to see is multiple cups in a larger area. Applying multiple cups in an area can treat organ function for several organs, treat an entire channel, etc.

You may have seen large clusters of cups on the upper back to treat wind invasions or clusters of cups on the lower back. Both of these are very common to see in clinic.

METHOD 1: STATIC CUPPING

Static cupping means applying the cups to the target points/areas and leaving them in place. This is what was described in Chapter 14.

The process is basic. Apply a light coat of oil, apply the cups, let them sit for the appropriate amount of time, remove them. This process can be repeated a couple of times, re-positioning the cups to get full coverage of the small diamond shaped areas between the cups that weren't treated on the first application.

Weak cupping

Weak or light cupping is considered to be tonifying. In weak cupping, the cups are applied with a light suction. To get a light suction, use a less intense flame. The flame is strongest right after it is lit, so you can wait a moment for the flame to burn down and is less intense. You can also use a smaller cotton ball to produce a smaller flame.

The amount of flesh drawn up into the cup should be very minimal – hardly raised. If it is too much you can press at where the skin and the lip of the cup meet to allow some air into the cup to reduce the suction. The patient should feel no discomfort, no pain, no sensation of pulling inside the cups.

Light cupping like this causes the skin to redden slightly rather than making deep bruises or blisters.

When to use weak cupping
Weak cupping is gentle and can be used anywhere on the body. This method stimulates movement of Qi and tonifies Qi and Blood without depleting the body. Because of its' action and because it doesn't bruise or blister at any point, it is suitable for a number of applications.

- Debilitated patients
  People who are constitutionally weak, have been through a long illness, have depleted Qi and Blood, etc. If you see deficiency, this method might be what you're looking for.

- Elderly patients
  Watch for very dry skin in the elderly and sometimes in the debilitated patients too. Dry skin will cause the cups to release faster than you'd like. Use more oil to fix this.

- Young children
  Especially those under the age of 7. Kids younger than seven have more fragile skin and need less stimulation, so weak cupping is great for them.

- On the face
  Weak cupping will not bruise, so you could use it on the face, *but* I would recommend pneumatic cups. Western patients get pretty nervous if you start getting flames close to their faces. The thin walled glass cups with the suction bulb on the top work well here.

Medium cupping
This is generally what you are doing when you are applying cupping. This method is also considered to be tonifying.

If the person you are treating is not debilitated and has a decent energy level, this will tonify the patient. Even so, *never* leave the cups on longer than 20 minutes because this *will* deplete your patient.

The flame is bigger for this level of suction and the cup is held close to the body when burning the oxygen out of the cup. You will see the skin pulled up further into the cup and it starts to look red fairly quickly.

Medium cupping can be applied almost anywhere on the body, but I might recommend lighter suction for the face unless you are treating something like Bells Palsy. And again for the face, be aware that western patients aren't fond of flames near their face and eyes. Might use a pneumatic or silicone cup on the face.

Medium cupping will work well for hot and cold bi syndromes, tonifying and moving Blood and Qi.

Strong cupping

This method is draining to the body, so you have to be sure your patient's condition is suitable for this method! The Wei Qi is most affected by this method. Pulse, tongue, and all s/sx should point to an Shi (excess or full) condition before you do this.

To use this method, you need a big fire. Use a larger cotton ball (you may have to combine two of them) and as soon as you soak and ignite it, get it into the cup to produce a strong vacuum. The skin will pretty quickly turn red and then purple inside the cup.

The skin will probably bruise and it can take up to 2 weeks for the bruise to resolve. During this time it is generally not tender or sensitive like when you whack your shin on the coffee table in the middle of the night, but it will be discolored during this time.

When to use strong cupping

When there is an excess condition and the person is not debilitated you can sue this. It affects Wei Qi strongly, moves Blood and Qi to address stagnation, and eliminates internal and external pathogenic factors.

This method is effective for hot bi syndromes and for frozen shoulder syndromes.

Cautions:

- Because this is a very draining method, leave cups on no longer than 10 minutes on the first application. You can leave them on up to 20 minutes in future applications.

- Be aware that this will break the small capillaries and the bruising will be noticeable. If your patient is going to or participating in an image sensitive event (weddings, beauty pageants, modeling gigs, etc.), they need to know this and make a decision accordingly as to whether they want you to do this at this time.

- This method is the one that is most likely to leave blisters on the skin.

- Don't use strong cupping on the face, stomach, abdomen, on the elderly and/or frail, on kids less than 14 years of age, or pregnant patients.

METHOD 2: FLASH CUPPING

This is also called empty cupping and shan guan fa in Chinese medical literature. It is a tonifying method. It is almost exclusively applied to the back of the body, never the face.

Flash cupping is applying a cup to the skin with either medium or strong suction, leaving the cup in place for a very short time (less than a minute), then repeatedly applying the cup in the same basic place multiple times. This is appropriate for older people and places where the cup won't stay on (due to body hair, the shape of the area, very loose skin, etc.). It is also appropriate when cold or heat pathogens are present in weak, frail, and elderly patients, as well as in children less than 14 years of age.

Flash cupping is also good for areas of skin numbness, deficiency, and hypo-function. The fire will warm the area and stimulate/move Qi and Blood and without stressing the body.

Be aware that repeatedly applying fire to a single cup will make the thing very hot! I rotate through 4 or 5 cups when I do this in a very small area or only on one point so that I don't burn the patient or myself.

You can also apply up to 12 cups at a time, leave them on for less than 60 seconds, then remove them starting with the first one you applied. You can repeat this for between 5 and 10 minutes during a session or until very slight bruising appears on the body. These bruises should fade within a couple of days.

METHOD 3: SLIDING CUPPING

This is my favorite method; I love doing this. Sliding cupping is also called moving cupping or tui guan fa in Chinese medical literature. It's often used for musculoskeletal pain and tightness in the upper back, lower back, shoulders, and sciatic pain areas. Patients that have this kind of pain and tightness usually love this modality. This is like a mixture of cupping, gua sha, and massage, but the massage is pulling not pushing. It feels fantastic.

This is a *draining* method. As a mater of fact, it's probably the *most* draining of all the methods we are talking about. Your patient should therefore be fairly strong energetically. This is also considered to be the most uncomfortable method of cupping. If your patient is currently or constitutionally weak this won't be fun for them and will actually drain them further.

This method is appropriate for larger areas and for areas of heavy musculature such as the upper back, lower back, thighs, and lateral thighs. It is usually applied to the 1st and 2nd Bladder channel lines when excess conditions such as heat and Qi and Blood stagnation. It is also used in some neurological conditions like post-stroke weakness, hemiplegia, or paralysis.

Here's how:
1. Oil the skin more than you normally would so that the cup will slide easily over the skin.

Order of sliding vs. static cups

If you are going to do both sliding and static cupping in a single session, *do the sliding cupping first*, then apply the static cups.

Once the static cups have been on a few minutes they leave big divots that persist for a while and are very hard to slide over.

2. Select a medium sized cup with smooth even edges. No sharp edges, chips, or cuts on the cup at all.

3. Apply a medium suction to the cup and immediately test it by gently trying to move it around. If the suction is too

weak it will pop off. If it's too strong it will hurt and won't move easily when you attempt movement. If you let the cup sit still too long it will make divots in the skin and be very hard to move. Be sure you do this quickly as soon as you suction it on to the skin!

4. Grip the cup in your dominant hand and use your non-dominant hand to support the skin around the cup and hold it still.

5. Pull and slide the cup along the meridian using long strokes. Short up and down strokes hurt! The point of this is to manipulate the excess energy in the area by bringing the heat this causes up to the surface of the skin.

    One of my instructors, the fabulous Dr. Xiaotian Shen, taught me to roll my wrist around in small circles while simultaneously moving the cup up and down the channel. Patients with muscle tightness and pain *love* this method and it doesn't hurt on the skin.

6. As you slide the cups around you will inevitably let a little air into the cup. It's not unusual to need to re-apply the cup a few times during sliding cupping.

The more internal heat that is present (whether that's heat from a pathogenic invader or heat from stagnation), the faster bruises will appear. This is very similar to what you are doing with gua sha (see Chapter 10).

The speed and depth of the bruising can be viewed diagnostically:
   • Deep, dark bruises that appear quickly can indicate a full or excess condition and/or an acute condition.
   • Light bruising can indicate empty or xu conditions.

Cautions

Besides the cautions already listed, add these:

- Don't use on open wounds, lesions or sunburns. Oddly, moving cupping is great for psoriasis, eczema, and acne, but you still can't do it right over the lesions.
- Don't use on children under 14 years of age.
- Don't use for weak, frail, or debilitated patients.
- The 1st treatment should be no more than 5 minutes. Successive treatments can be longer, but never more than 15 minutes.
- Never use this method on the face or front of the body. Use Bladder channel points on the back to address problems in these areas instead.
- The same is true for Bi syndromes. Don't apply it on the painful point directly, but you can use it *near* the area if there is enough musculature beneath it.

METHOD 4: NEEDLING AND CUPPING

Also a draining method, this form of cupping is most often used or hot Bi syndromes (like arthritis where the joint is hot and painful, even feels hot when you hold the back of your hand to it) and for wind damp cold type Bi syndromes. You will find this most commonly on the knees and elbows. Needling the area then applying cupping can be an effective way to drain the excess heat, wind, cold, or damp and stop the pain in the joint.

Since this method can cause the needle to penetrate further into the body than acupuncture alone, **you *really need your instructor's guidance here!!***

To use this method, you would:

1. Apply a ½ to 1 cun acupuncture needle to the area you are treating.

2. Apply a cup on top of that needle using a medium to strong application for joints and a weak to medium suction if over a muscular area. You have to be sure the cup is tall enough to accommodate the height of the needle.
3. Retain for 10-15 minutes

Cautions
- This method is *not* recommended for back shu points nor on the chest! There are too many vital organs close to the surface here.
- You might consider using a bamboo cup in this method because of the height of the cups. If you have a glass cup that will work, you can do that too. (Just between us, I've also used small/tall jars for this. I bought a small jar of olives that turned out to be perfect for this after I'd put all of those olives on a pizza or three. I always prefer glass jars I can see through.)
- Not recommended for kids of any age.

METHOD 5: BLOODLETTING AND CUPPING

As this method is clearly a draining method (like literally!), it is only appropriate for healthy adults with excess conditions! This method is also called full cupping, bleeding cupping, and xue guan fa in Chinese medical literature. It looks an awful lot like the hijama wet cupping method in Arabic medical treatments.

Bleeding cupping is appropriate for sudden rises in blood pressure (people who've never had high blood pressure before but suddenly develop it), for pus discharge, for blood heat conditions, and Qi/Blood stagnations.

Though you can apply this to many points on the body, the most common application is at Du 14, the strongest Yang point in the body and the one that can release the most heat. To apply bleeding cupping here:

1. Position the patient so they are laying face down with their head in a face cradle, or sitting in a chair and leaning forward comfortably with the face and head supported by a pillow.

2. Use a plum blossom needle at Du 14 with a strong enough tapping method to cause bleeding.

3. Immediately apply a large cup with strong suction over Du 14. You will see the blood come up more quickly into the cup. If you caused enough bleeding, you will get somewhere between 30ml (2 tbsp) and 60ml (about ¼ of a cup) of blood in the cup.

4. When you remove the cup you will need your blood spill kit handy. Glove up and use a lot of paper towels at the opening when you release the cup. Be sure to release it *away from your face!*

You might think this is going to be a messy blood bath, but it won't be. The blood usually coagulates into a weird gelatinous blob in the cup before you even remove it.

Cautions
*   Not for use on kids, elderly, or debilitated patients!
*   *Never* for people on anti-coagulants!
*   *Never* more than 100ml at a time
*   Don't do this more than once a month
*   Use all the standard blood borne disease precautions when you are doing this.
*   *Never* on large blood vessels because that causes too much bleeding.

There are several other methods of cupping you might want to be aware of, but which are not commonly used in western acupuncture clinics very often. Sometimes these are too much work to cram into a single one-hour treatment, sometimes it's because of insurance or legal constraints.

Fire throwing and cotton attaching methods

These are actually kind of bad ass to use, but can scare the hell out of a western patient base. I've still done it. It works really well and can be very effective.

This method is used on the lateral sides of the body or on the back with the patient sitting up right. In the fire throwing method you light a small cotton ball and leave it inside a large cup when you attach it to the body. The oxygen burns out quickly and causes a very strong suction.

In the cotton attaching method, you soak a small amount of sterile gauze in alcohol, stick it on the inside of a large cup, light it on fire and attach it to the body. Same kind of a deal as the fire throwing method. I actually like the cotton attaching method better. I attach it at the far end of the cup from the opening using my forceps so that it is as far from the skin as possible, light a cotton ball like I normally do and use that to light the gauze on fire, then quickly put it on the body. I also use a cute potholder mitt on my dominant hand so I don't burn myself when I apply it.

The big caution here besides (duh) fire near the skin is you absolutely *never never never* apply this like you would a normal cup with the patient lying face down. This is always done on the side of the body so that the flame cannot accidentally fall onto the skin.

Moxa cupping

This is also called hot needle cupping and ai guan fa. It is a tonification method that combines moxibustion and cupping and needling. It also takes a lot of practice. You insert a metal handled needle, put a moxa ball on top of it like you would for hot needle therapy, let the moxa burn out, safely shake off the ash, and *then* apply a cup on top of the area. The needle stays hot, even though the moxa is gone. This is a method for treating cold syndromes of the Spleen and Stomach, for lower back pain that is coming from a Kidney Yang deficiency/xu cold, and for bed wetting or impotence caused by deficient cold.

Herbal cupping

This method combines herbal medicine with bamboo cupping. The bamboo cups are boiled in the herbal formula for about 30 minutes, then cooled *just* enough not to burn the skin. You apply the cup like you normally would. The herbal formula is transferred to the cup which then transfers it to the body when the cup is applied. Awesome for wind damp cold invasions with aching and stiffness in the neck and upper back. Works well for common cold, asthma, and coughing. But you can see how labor intensive this is and what care it would take not to burn the patient or yourself with the fire or steam. And of course, you have to own a bamboo cupping set.

CHAPTER 16
Precautions and Aftercare for Cupping

We have covered a lot of the precautions, contraindications, and "gotcha" things that can happen in cupping, but there are a few more to know or re-emphasize.

SIGNED INFORMED CONSENT

I've said it before, but it bears repeating. Always tell your patient what is going to happen, what the risks are, and what you are going to do to avoid them as much as is within your power. You don't have to scare the bejesus out of them, but you can explain in a calm, confident manner what's going on. Be sure your informed consent forms are signed and that they explain the risks and possible marks on the body that will result.

BLISTERS

I do a lot of cupping, but have only seen blisters come up a couple of times. Hypersensitive patients are more likely to get them. Patients whose cups are left on too long can get them too. If you are paying attention and stay in the room with your patient you are much less likely to see bad blistering.

Small blisters

These happen once in a while regardless of the precautions you take and how much you are paying attention. Hypersensitive patients are the more likely candidates for these. Small blisters will reabsorb into the body within a couple of days and are no real cause for concern. Make a note of the occurrence in the patient's chart and be aware of this for the next treatment. Let the patient know they are there and that they will reabsorb within a couple of days.

Large and severe blisters

These are likely to occur if the cups are left on too long. Drain these with a sterile acupuncture needle and cover them with gauze to prevent infection. Send the patient home with some of the miracle Chinese burn cream. . . I mean Ching Wan Hung. . . and tell them to apply it several times per day and keep the blisters covered.

If this happens on your watch, give them an unopened tube of this stuff. Engender goodwill as much as you can.

AFTERCARE

Though some schools don't teach aftercare for cupping, I feel it is important. Cupping 'opens' the body to release toxins and pathogens for about 24 hours after the treatment. This means that toxins and pathogens can come *in* as well.

I encourage my patients to keep the area covered for 24 hours, even if it's only with a shirt or light scarf. I also tell them to avoid very hot showers or baths, hot tubs, very cold showers and baths, and to avoid heavy work afterwards.

This is an important precaution because patients with musculoskeletal pain often feel terrific afterwards and are eager to go do all the things they couldn't do when they felt crappy. This will further deplete the body and they will feel bad again.

Give them the precautions and after care instructions, preferably in writing, so they understand why you are saying what you are. If you put it in writing they are more likely o remember what to do and what not to do.

I hate it when medical professionals blast a bunch of verbal cautions and aftercare stuff at me. There's no way I'm going to remember it. Neither will your patients.

SECTION 6
Electroacupuncture

Electroacupuncture, also called EA and e-stim, is a bloody brilliant combination of a metal handled acupuncture needle and a very mild electrical current. EA was developed in China in the 1930's as a way to get more stimulation time on more needles without the practitioner needing to manually stimulate the needles.

This section takes a look at EA basics, using the AWQ-104L electroacupuncture device as the major example. You can apply the principles you learn here about frequency, intensity, and wave patterns to any model. Also covered are safety precautions, methods of use, and treatment patterns.

This page intentionally left blank.

CHAPTER 17
Electroacupuncture Basics

Acupuncture treatment start much the same way: interview the patient, decide on a diagnosis and differentiation, craft a treatment plan, then insert the appropriate needles and manually stimulate them to get a Qi reaction.

The difference here is that you have *also* selected sites to which you would like to apply electroacupuncture (EA or e-stim). Electrodes are attached to these needles and stimulation is applied.

BASIC PRINCIPLES

I could just tell you how to attach the wires, what settings to adjust, and how long to leave it on. But any fool can do that. That's just a technical how-to. You are studying to be an *artist*, a professional who knows stuff and makes wise decisions. And to be that person, you have to know how and why stuff works so that you can use your skills confidently and know what to do when something isn't working right.

So with that in mind, here are some simple basic principles about how electricity works, how it interacts with a human body, and how that e-stim machine works that you have in your hand.

Positive (+) and negative (-)

Electricity and the flow of electrical current works based on certain rules. This is true whether it's flowing in your house or through that EA machine you're learning about.
Electrical current needs a way to flow and a way to exit before it functions for you. You might compare this to the

way your plumbing works. Let's say you have a sink full of dirty dishes and need to get them clean. You have to turn on the flow of water to wash the dishes, but it's equally important that you have a way to drain that water away.

When you are talking about electricity the same basic idea applies. You need the electrical current to flow in, but you also need somewhere for it to exit. The term used for the current going to target area is positive (+) current. The current going away from or flowing back to the source is the negative (–) current. When there is both a + and a – connected correctly, this is called a "closed circuit."

This is what you are going for when you apply electroacupuncture – a closed circuit.

Closed circuits

EA units have wires that go from the unit to the needles. The end attaching to the e-stim unit will either look like a headphone jack or they will have a proprietary ends. This end is attached to a double wire.

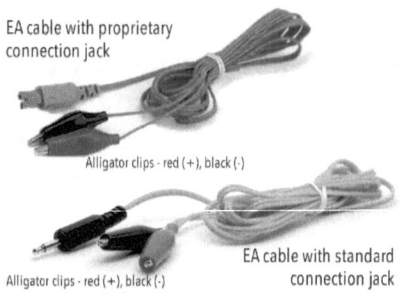

EA cable with proprietary connection jack

Alligator clips - red (+), black (-)

Alligator clips - red (+), black (-)

EA cable with standard connection jack

The opposite end of the cable is splits into two wires near the end and then ends in alligator clips that are either red or black. The red end is the positive (+) end of the circuit. The black end is the negative (–) end of the circuit.

How far it flows

Electricity only flows so far before it loses strength and becomes ineffective for our purposes. Most of us don't really have to be aware of that. We turn on light switches and the light comes on. We plug in our phones and they start charging.

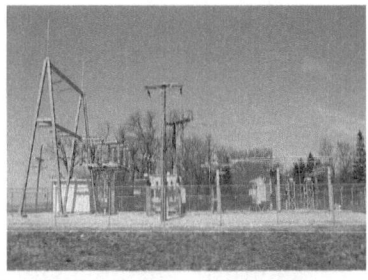

What you might or might not know is that where that power is generated and where you are using it can be a *long* distance apart. Your power company has to do some pretty big stuff to keep it flowing in a useable manner across these large distances. That's why you see electrical booster stations here and there. By the way, don't live close to these. Not great for your health.

What does all of this have to do with you?

There are two basic takeaways from the explanation above that apply to what you want to do with e-stim.

You need a closed circuit.

You need to attach both of those alligator clips so needles so that the e-stim works right. You usually attach both to needles, but I've seen come practitioners close the circuit by attaching the red clip to a needle and the black clip attached to a piece of wet gauze on the patient's skin somewhat near the needle with the red clip.

The black clip, the negative pole, is the strongest. Attach this clip to the primary point you want to stimulate. The red clip is the support wire that carries overflow current back and away. Place this clip on the secondary support point.

Proximity of the red clip to the black clip.

Because electricity only flows so far (and because you don't have a tiny booster station to place on the patient) you need to be aware that placing the ends (also referred to as negative and positive poles) too far apart will not give you the benefits you are looking for.

Conversely, putting the clips too *close* to each other is also undesirable. That concentrates the electrical stimulation too much and can cause pain. This also can "confuse" the area and the stimulation doesn't really end up where you need it.

So how close *do* you put them?

There's no guide really, but as a general rule, you want the poles no less than 6 cun apart. What is the maxiumum? That truly depends. I've never found a definitive answer – most of the time the answer is "not too far." Talk to your instructor about this!

Example:
OK, that said, let me give you an example from my clinic records. I've seen stuff like this often enough that I think this one is a good one to share with you.

> Let's say you have a patient who comes in with right side shoulder pain that is most intense just below the shoulder around LI 15 and this pain radiates downward on the arm. You palpate and find that the tenderness ends around the elbow at LI 11. You could needle both of these points then place the black clip on LI 15 since this is the most intense point of pain. Black is the negative side and contains the strongest current.

You would couple that with the red clip on LI 11, the secondary point. This completes the circuit and runs the current from the top of the painful area to the bottom.

What if the pain is equally distributed between LI 11 and LI 15? Then both of these points would be primary pain points. You want to give the primary stimulation to both of these points during the treatment session. You could do these in reverse, but as an example, place the black clip on LI 15 and the red on LI 11 and apply stimulation for 15 minutes. Then you could shut it all down and switch the clips, putting the black clip on LI 11 and the red on LI 15 for another 15 minutes.

Some e-stim units have a switch to change polarity (thus switching negative to positive and vice versa) so that you don't have to physically move the leads, but you still have to turn all the knobs to zero when you switch the polarity.

BENEFITS OF EA

I have a patient came up to me in the grocery store some time ago who wanted to introduce me to her husband. When she did she laughingly said, "This is the lady who stabs, shocks, and burns me every time I go to see her and it makes me feel great!"

That's how the general public sees us, folks! So given that we stab and burn people, why the heck would we want to add zapping people to that? There are some great reasons for this.

1. Hand fatigue
   You can stimulate pertinent points manually using rotation and the other methods you learned in the first

techniques book,[13] but if you need to do several of them that can get very time consuming and tiring.

2. Strength and time of stimulus
    EA can provide a continuous amount of stimulation for longer than you can. And it can provide a stronger stimulus without causing tissue damage. Twirling, lifting and thrusting will cause more damage than you want. *Could* you stimulate up to 6 points for 20 minutes during a single one hour treatment? Nope. Not even if you use both hands at the same time. . . which you can't. Not with any degree of reliability anyway. And sometimes you need a stronger stimulus than you could give by manual manipulation, like in cases of neuralgia and paralysis. EA can do that for you.

3. Better control
    It is so much easier to control frequency of stimulus and how much stimulus the needle gets with EA than it is by hand. Most EA machines have fluctuating wave patterns to choose from that you could probably not achieve reliably using manual methods.

Now with all that woohoo, I need to tell you there is a definitely downside or two as well. The big one is lack of direct participation on your part. Machines don't respond to minute changes that take place during treatment.

One example is that bodies get used to stimulation over a short period of time and learn to tune it out. When you apply EA and the patient feels the "buzz" of it, if you wait about 10 minutes and ask if they still feel it the answer will be no. A machine cannot know that it needs to adjust the stimulation a little bit,

---

[13] Calhoun, Catherine D., L.Ac. *Acupuncture Techniques 101: Safety, CNT, and Needling Techniques*, Cats TCM Notes Press. 2019. ISBN: 1070169552.

but you do because you have the ability to directly communicate with the patient.

Most of us apply needles, set the EA stimulation, then leave to attend to other patients. It's not an ideal situation – in a perfect world I would give the whole one hour to the patient – but it's how you stay in business as an acupuncturist and actually make a living. If you practice this way too, then "set it, adjust it, let the patient rest" works pretty well.

MATERIALS YOU NEED

Shortest list I've ever given you: you need an e-stim (EA) machine.

If you look on any acupuncture supplier site you will see an eye-crossing array of devices to choose from. I obviously cannot address the use of each one. I'll give you the basic principles in the following chapters, which you can apply to any EA device you like.

I use the AWQ-104L EA machine. I've owned one of these for years and I love it. FYI, I get no endorsement money from these

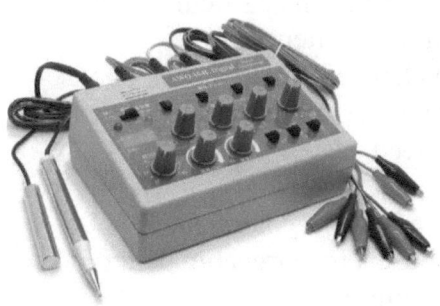

folks. I just like the machine a lot. Not only is it a workhorse that shows no signs of slowing down after many years of use, it has a good set of features that allows me to talk about several cool things you can do with an EA machine.

You can get these on LhasaOMS (who also does not pay me a dime to say that, by the way – just a good site with good prices) for around $250 USD, but they are frequently on sale.

That's a good chunk of money when you're a student, so you might save that purchase for after you graduate and start up your own clinic or acupuncture service since you can *generally* write that off on your taxes. . . .if you're in the USA, I mean. Given the administration when this was published, however. . . . who knows.

Here's what's cool about this machine:
1. It's got a great range of stimulation levels.
    You can take this anywhere from 1Hz up to 1,000Hz at the high range. When you use this below the level at which the patient can sense it, you can also get microcurrent effects.

2. You can stimulate up to 4 channels at a time.
    Each channel controls a pair of electrodes, meaning you can stimulate up to 8 needles at a time. *And* each pair is independently controlled so you get the effect you want in the area you want it in.

3. Three adjustable patterns of stimulation
    Different stimulation patterns are appropriate for different disease and syndromes. This particular unit gives you a continuous, an intermittent, and a dense/dispersed pattern to choose from and each one is easily adjustable to a pretty wide range so you get just the therapeutic effect you need.

And all that from a 9 volt battery. My battery lasts about 3 months with pretty heavy usage. I use a rechargeable battery and disconnect it after every use. Your mileage may vary!

Are there less expensive machines? Yep. I've used these two as well.

This one, the E-Stim II, worked well for a while and was inexpensive – I think I bought it for less than $100 right after I got licensed. It's got a little pulsing light that tells you how fast the stimulus is pulsing. The good stuff about it is that it's an inexpensive way to get started with e-stim. The downside is that it's only got 2 channels, only does 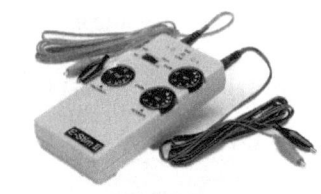 continuous stimulation rather than allowing you to regulate the wave dispersal pattern. . . . and it only lasted about a year before it literally melted down. I don't recommend it. Save your pennies and get something else.

The other one that I used a lot in student clinic and loved is this one: the ITS ES-130 unit. You can adjust the intensity and frequency on this unit, it's got the cool blinking light so you can see how fast the stim is hitting, but the wave pattern isn't adjustable here either. Nevertheless, it's a sturdy, high quality unit and I liked it a lot.

It's got three output channels, so you can stimulate up to 6 needles at a time. The connectors aren't universal though – they are proprietary. If one of the cables or alligator clips goes bad, you have to replace it with the proprietary kind. They cost a little more than the AWQ-104L – usually around $300 USD, but they are a great portable device that will fit in the palm of your hand, they last a long time, and they take a lot of use and abuse. Battery life is good too.

> **Bonus Fun Fact**
> Most TENS units like chiropractors sell for pain control come with wire leads that plug into the TENS unit with a small headphone type jack. The other end of the wire generally has some replaceable pads that stick on the skin.

Here's the fun fact part. You *can* replace *those* leads with a lead that has the little headphone jack looking end on one side and an alligator clip on the other. Now it can function as an e-stim machine for acupuncture. It works in a pinch, but I find the "zap" it gives feels sharper somehow. But it will work in a pinch. I still like the feel of an EA machine better.

INDICATIONS/FUNCTIONS FOR ELECTROACUPUNCTURE

EA is used for many different kinds of syndromes and disease conditions.

Syndrome	Examples
Pain syndromes	Trigeminal neuralgia, sciatica, pain in the occipital area, migraines, periarthritis of the shoulder, joint problems such as knee pain and tennis elbow, kidney pain, abdominal pain, pain in scar tissues. It's even been used to help heal broken bones. Protocol for all of these coming later.
Flaccidity syndromes	Paraplegia, hemiplegia, facial paralysis.
Organ syndromes	Gastric spasms, biliary colic, renal colic, dysmenorrhea.

There have been studies in China on cancer patients who received e-stim therapy for four weeks, 5 times per week for a total of a 20 treatment course, whose T-cells and killer cells increased by 15% after treatment.

Moral to the story: this is good stuff.

CHAPTER 18
Electroacupuncture Methods

To use electroacupuncture, you need to select good quality, metal handled needles for you're the points in your treatment where you intend to apply EA (meaning you can use other types of needles in places you don't want to apply EA).

At the beginning, an EA treatment looks like any other acupuncture treatment: patient interview, determine diagnosis and differentiation, make a treatment plan based on the diagnosis and differentiation, insert the appropriate needles, get the Qi reaction (also called "De Qi" in a lot of literature). After you've done this, *then* you can apply e-stim to the points you have identified as pertinent for this modality for this patient at this time.

Here's a *general* overview about what happens after the needles are in and the de qi has arrived.

1. Get out e-stim machine and attach the battery.
   Most e-stim machines run on 9-volt batteries. I find the batteries last much longer if you disconnect them after each use and reconnect them right before you use them. This also keeps the batteries from leaking and corroding the attachments when not in use.

2. Attach the leads to the machine.
   The leads are the long double wires with a jack that attaches to the EA machine on one end and alligator clips on the other ends after the cable splits.

   I've shown two different types of cables here. One has a

squarish looking end that attaches to the e-stim unit. This is a proprietary style used on the ITO ® ES-130. The other cable pictured is more standard, using what

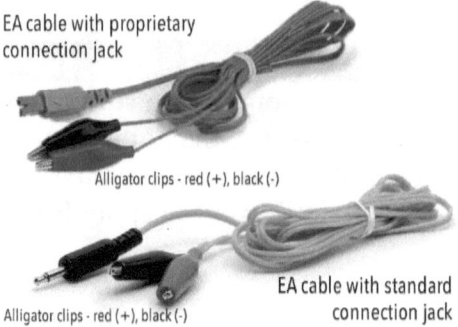

EA cable with proprietary connection jack

Alligator clips - red (+), black (-)

Alligator clips - red (+), black (-)

EA cable with standard connection jack

looks like a headphone jack to attach to the EA unit. It also has alligator clips on the opposite ends.

3. Attach the leads to the selected points.
    Follow all EA treatment protocol guidelines and precautions for point selection and placement of leads. See the precaution and tips section at the end of this chapter as well as the guidelines in the last chapter about how far apart to place the stimulation points.

    .

    Make sure the unit is off when you do this and that the leads are attached to the EA unit. Press on the red or black plastic sleeve over the alligator clip to open the clip. Place the alligator clip of the handle of a metal-handled needle and release your grip to allow the clip to attach to the needle.

    Do this gently so that you don't move the needle around much. You may need to do some adjusting to keep this comfortable. The weight of the clip and the wire can bend the needle. I often tuck the wire under the patient a little so that it doesn't fall on the floor and yank on the needle.

4. Set the intensity.
    a. Make sure all dials are set to zero and the unit's power is OFF at this point.
    b. Set the frequency to a medium range before you turn the unit on, but all other dials are still set to zero.
    c. Power the unit on.
    d. Very, very slowly, in hair-fine increments, increase the intensity. Ask the patient for the following feedback.
        i. Ask them to tell you when they can *just barely* feel the stimulation. Tell them you are going to keep increasing it.
        ii. Ask them to tell you when it feels strong. Tell them you are going to go just a little more.
        iii. Ask the patient to tell you when it is getting too strong.

    Back off of that setting just a little and make sure it feels strong but within the patient's comfort level.

5. Set the frequency
    You begin in step 4 with setting the frequency to a medium level so that the patient can easily give you feedback about the intensity. Now you want to reset the frequency for the best result for the patient's disease condition or syndrome.

    It is possible that the frequency required to best treat your patient is faster than the medium setting you started with. This might cause patient discomfort. If it does, adjust the *intensity* setting to a lower number.

6. Set the waveform
   Not all machines have this adjustment option. If yours
   does, you can choose the waveform that gives the best
   therapeutic result for your patient's current
   disease/syndrome. If it does not, no worries.

7. Kill a couple of minutes in an efficient manner.
   Talk with the patient a few moments, explaining that the
   sensation might disappear in a short time and making
   sure everything is currently comfortable for them. Put
   on some music. If it's chilly, put a TDP lamp on their
   feet or put a sheet or light blanket over them. (I have
   some yoga blocks in my office I use to strategically keep
   the sheet or blanket off of the needles for a more
   comfortable rest.)

   All of this time-killing gives the e-stim sensations time
   to settle in their bodies. Ask if they can still feel the
   sensation of the EA.
   a. If the answer is no, adjust the *intensity* slightly
      until they can feel it again and that the sensation
      is definitely noticeable but within their comfort
      tolerance. You can leave the frequency and
      waveform settings just as they are.
   b. If the answer is yes, make sure it feels strong but
      comfortable to them, then lower the lights and
      step out.

8. Check in during treatment
   Because the body tends to get used to the EA sensations
   and tune them out, check back a couple of times during
   the treatment to be sure the patient can still feel them. If
   they cannot, increase the *intensity* setting slightly until
   they can.

   Needle retention time is usually no more than 20

minutes for e-stim.

9. Ending the EA
   At the end of the treatment, turn all of the
   electroacupuncture machine's knobs down to zero
   (starting with the intensity setting) and then power the
   machine off.

   Gently remove the leads from the needles and put the
   machine and leads away, remembering to remove the
   connections to the battery.

10. Final stuff
    Remove patients' needles, schedule the following
    session for them, and send them home with any aftercare
    instructions they might need.

INTENSITY, FREQUENCY, WAVEFORM

There are three big things to understand about electrical
stimulation of an acupuncture point and all machines have this
in some form or terminology or another. TENS units might call
waveform a "burst pattern," for instance.

Intensity

This is *how strong* the stimulation is. Intensity adjustments
are often from 1 (low or very weak) to 10 (high or very
strong).

Frequency

The "bzzzz" or pulse of electricity you feel from an EA
machine or TENS unit isn't constant, but stimulates then
stops and repeats over and over until you disconnect the
power.

Frequency is *how often* the patient feels the stimulation. Pulse frequency can be adjusted on most machines from very slow to so fast that it *feels* constant.

Waveform

Every machine has a waveform of some kind, even if it's a simple on/off pattern that you can't adjust. Nothing at all wrong with that: that's the standard in China and they use it with great effect. Some machines have a broader range of on/off/intensity/strength bursts for different applications, but you can absolutely practice well without the fancy schmancy stuff.

If the machine you are using offers a waveform adjustment, be sure to set the intensity knob back to zero before you change the waveform pattern. After you change the pattern, gradually increase the intensity again.

Don't place pairs too close together

Don't place the positive and negative pairs too close together. We talked about that already.

Don't cross the body

Don't cross from one side of the body to the other with a single pair of leads!

Place a single black/red pair on the *same* side of the body. Crossing from one side to the other with a single pair can interfere with the electrical activity in the heart and mess with the heart rhythm. You *definitely* don't want to do this. Always place the pairs on the same side of the body.

Can you place one pair on one side and another pair on another side of the body? Yes, you can. In the illustration here you can see a single negative/positive pair on the right side of the 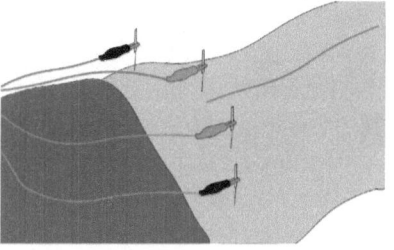 back (green wires) and another pair on the left side of the back (blue wires). That's ok.

Handle, not the shaft

Always attach the clip to the metal *handle* of the needle. Never attach it to the shaft! This can weaken the needle and cause a needle break.

If you Google images for acupuncture e-stim you will see crazy people who attach the clips to the shaft of the needle. No. Fail. Don't do this. Even if some goofy chiropractor or PT puts out a Youtube video about it doesn't mean they know what the hell they are doing. They don't get nearly as much education about this as you do. Don't use them as a guide. You know more.

Increase intensity gradually

Turn stimulation intensity up very gradually and carefully. This is not just a comfort measure. Sudden increases in the intensity can cause an intense musculature contraction which can bend and break needles.

Intensity stimulation should never approach the level of pain!

Caution near spine and brain

When applying e-stim near the spine or brain, intensity should always be mild.

Caution near the heart

When applying e-stim on the chest and back near the region of the heart *do not cross the body with a single pair of leads* to avoid messing with the electrical activity of the heart. As a matter of fact, just don't ever cross from one side of the body to the other with a pair. Never.

Other patient population cautions

- Be extremely cautious in patients with heart disease, seizures, or who are pregnant.

- Be very cautious in patients who are elderly and weak.

- Be cautious with patients who have metal implants. Don't touch the implant with the needle at all.

Contraindications

- Do not use EA for patients with pacemakers or any other electric implants (insulin pumps, pain regulators, etc).

- Personally, I think using EA with patients with seizure disorders should be a contraindication. But that's just me.

- Never cross the body with a single pair of leads. Never.

This page intentionally left blank.

CHAPTER 19
Treatment Protocols and Point Selections

There are five basic ways to treat with electroacupuncture:
1. According to nerve distribution
2. According to channel distribution
3. According to Zangfu relationships
4. According to local point reactivity
5. According to disease

ACCORDING TO NERVE DISTRIBUTION

Stimulating according to the pathway of the nerves is a lovely way to address pain, numbness, paralysis/partial paralysis, and flaccidity syndromes.

I recommend you look up the nerve pathways and try to plot the acupuncture points that are around and on them to get a better feel for how this works. Once you have done that, select points that are close to the nerve pathway for best effect.

Let's talk about nerve distribution in various the areas of the body and the commonly treated points along those nerve pathways.

Head

You can use these points to treat trigeminal neuralgia (TN), Bells Palsy, and various forms of facial paralysis.

Use mild stimulation on the head rather than strong stimulation, regardless of the strength of the condition. Use very mild stimulation for Bells Palsy if you catch it very early, but once it stabilizes you can strengthen stimulation.

For facial paralysis, wait a week after the onset so that the body stabilizes. Then you can begin stimulation and even use stronger stimulation if the patient can tolerate it.

Remember that you need a pair of points for stimulation to work. You can always use St 7 as your secondary point to treat the trigeminal nerves, as this is right around where the TN splits into the three branches.

Nerve	Points commonly selected
Facial nerve	Treating the facial nerve can treat Bells Palsy and other forms of facial paralysis and flaccidity. • Sj 17 • Qian zheng This is an extra point ½ to 1 cun anterior to the earlobe.
Trigeminal nerve	The trigeminal nerve has 3 branches: the ophthalmic branch going to the forehead and eye area, the maxillary branch going to the temples and sinus areas and upper jaw, and the mandibular branch supplying the lower jaw and side of the face/ear. These branches can be used to treat trigeminal neuralgia and other forms of facial pain/dysfunction. • Opthalmic branch: Use Gb 14, Bl 2 • Maxillary branch: St 2 • Mandibular branch: St 7, Jia Cheng Jiang (extra point below the lower lip

Upper limbs

The cervical and upper thoracic Jiaji points are often used as a way to treat the upper limbs. The Jiaji points sit ½ cun lateral from the centerline of the spine. They are located right over the nerve junctions between the spinal and peripheral nerves.

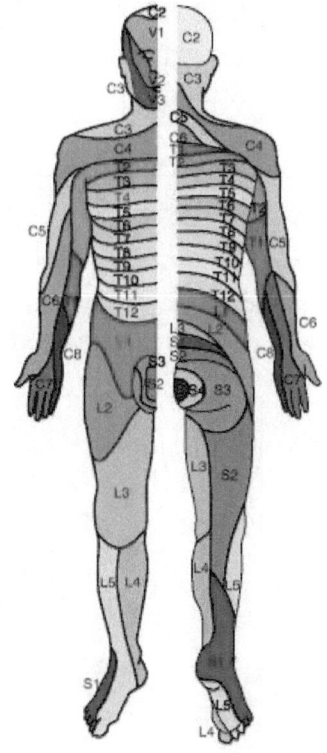

The peripheral nerves transmit both motor and sensory information between the limbs and the brain, which means you can treat these points to affect the limbs. Note on number/letter combinations on the illustration to the right. These correspond to the cervical, thoracic, lumbar, and sacral bones and peripheral nerves. The left side of the illustration is the anterior of the body; the right side represents the posterior side of the body.

By applying EA to these areas you can affect the areas you need to treat without directly treating them. By applying electroacupuncture to the cervical Jiaji point at C7, for instance, you could treat pain, numbness, and tingling in the index, middle fingers, and palm.

You can also use regular points that are close to the affected nerves for treatment instead of or in addition to the Jiaji points.

Nerve	Points commonly selected
Ulnar nerve	• Ht 2, SI 18, Jiaji Ht 2 is right on the ulnar nerve
Radial nerve	The radial nerve starts at the back on the scapula, then curves around the arm and innervates the fingers. • LI 13, LI 11, Jiaji
Median nerve	• Pc 3, Pc 4, Pc 6, Jiaji

Lower limbs

Jiaji points can be used to treat lower limb problems just like they can be used to treat upper limb problems.

Nerve	Points commonly selected
Sciatic nerve	This is actually a bundle of nerves that begins as individual peripheral nerves that bunch together in the lower back and travel through the gluteus muscles. The sciatic nerve bundle splits into three branches: one innervates the anterior thigh, another the lateral leg, and the final one innervates the posterior aspect of the leg. • Gb 30 – this is a point that treats most things sciatica. You can use this as a primary or secondary point for pain on any of the three sciatic branches. • Posterior side sciatic pain Huan Zhong and Bl 37– Huan zhong an extra point between Gb 30 and Du 2 you can use for sciatic pain down the posterior aspect of the leg. Couple it with Bl 37, also on the posterior midline of the leg. • Lateral side sciatic pain Gb 30 and Gb 34 work well together for this. • Anterior thigh sciatic pain Gb 30 and St 36 can be a good combination for pain that wraps from the gluteal muscles to the anterior thigh.
Tibial nerve	Bl 40 treats tibial nerve problems

Nerve	Points commonly selected
Common peroneal nerve	Gb 34 and Ling hou (extra point)
Lumbar nerves	Use Bl 23, 24, and 25
Sacral nerves	Use Bl 31-34

ACCORDING TO CHANNEL DISTRIBUTION

Pain often follows channels. Back pain on the upper back, for instance, will often follow the Bladder channel, so you can treat key points along the Bladder channel and relieve the pain. Even the sciatica example above could be addressed this way: posterior sciatic pain correlates to the lower Bladder channel, lateral sciatic pain to the Gallbladder channel, and anterior sciatic pain to the Stomach channel.

Treating according to channel distribution goes beyond just treatment of pain, however. You could treat digestive dysfunction by treating the Stomach and/or Spleen channel, for instance.

ACCORDING TO ZANGFU ORGAN RELATIONSHIP

One example is to treat back shu points to address organ problems. Kidney xu could be treated by applying e-stim at Bl 23, the back shu of the Kidney.

SELECTION OF LOCAL POINTS

I gave an example in the Chapter 17 about LI 15 and LI 11 on the lateral arm. This would be an example of using local points to treat problems in that local area. The pain was in this area, those points were the most tender, so they got the e-stim.

You will learn more about this in your treatment of disease studies, but this is a quick starter pack.

Disease condition	Points commonly selected
Facial paralysis	• Qian zheng, Sj 17, Gb 14, Bl 2, St 2, Jia cheng jiang • St 4, St 6, Gb 20, Li 4
Trigeminal neuralgia	• Gb 14, Bl 2, St 2, Jia cheng jiang, St 7 • LI 4, Lv 2, Gb 20 Lv 2 treats Liver wind, which is one of the culprits causing TN.
Sciatic pain	• Lumbar Jiaji, Bl 23, Bl 24, Bl 25, Bl 31, Bl 32 Gb 30, Bl 36, Bl 37, Bl 40, Gb 34, Bl 57, Bl 60, St 31, St 38 Use the stomach points for anterior branch sciatic pain. Works well with a dense or dense/disperse wave form (see below).
Hemiplegia	• St 12, Ht 2, Si 8, Pc 3, Pc 6, LI 13, LI 11, Gb 30, Bl 37, Bl 40, Gb 34, Ling Hou • Gb 20, Bl 10, Gb 21, Li 15, Li 4, Sj 5, Bl 60, Lv 2 You can use any of these. Works well with disperse and continuous waveforms. See below. Use a gentle stimulation for paralyzed patients – watch for the first signs of muscle twitch and stop there.
Arthritis	Local points. Treat according to affected joints. Select corresponding nerve points. Use a dense or dense/disperse wave pattern. By the way, you can use this method with artificial knees and hips. Just don't touch the needle to the metal implants.

Disease condition	Points commonly selected
Toothache	• Jia Cheng Jiang, Sj 17 • St 6, St 7, Gb 20, Li 4, St 44
Schizophrenia (also treats insomnia)	• Primary points: Du 24, Du 20, Du 16, Gb 20 • Use the appropriate ones that apply to your patient's diagnosis and differentiation: Ht 7, Pc 6, Li 4, Li 11, Gb 34, ST 40
Obesity	• Primary points: St 25, Sp 15, ST 31, St 34, Li 15, Li 14 • Points that stimulate the metabolism and treat phlegm retention: St 36, St 40, Sp 9, Li 11 If fat is mostly in the abdominal area (central obesity), choose stomach and abdominal points. You can use the lower limb points to stimulate the metabolism.

If you have the luxury of having a machine on which you can select different waveform patterns you can refine your treatment a bit. There are four basic waveforms that you can vary with some machines.

Dense wave

This is the wave pattern that comes with all EA machines, including the non-adjustable machines. The visual

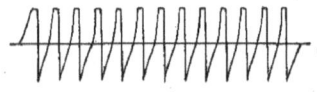

representation looks like the one to the right. You can guess from the visual that this fluctuates fairly rapidly and regularly between a higher and lower pulse and is generally adjustable between 50 and 100 pulses per second.

Functions and indications:

- Calming and tranquilizing effect.
- Inhibits sensory and motor nerves.
- Relieves pain, tranquilizes the mind, relieves spasms of the muscles and blood vessels.

Disperse/Sparse wave

While the previous wave pattern was a high frequency pattern, this one is a low frequency pattern, pulsing between 2 and 5 times per second. This pattern has a more activating function, so can be good for people recovering from stroke or injury.

Functions and indications:

- Induces muscular contraction and enhances the tension of muscles and ligaments.
- Treats paralysis, muscle injuries, ligaments and joints (especially for stressed and stretched or flaccid tissues).

Dense-disperse/Sparse wave

This waveform combines and alternates the dense wave and the sparse wave patterns above. Each 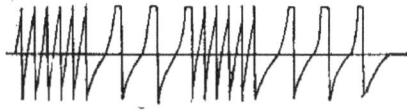 pattern lasts about a second and a half before alternating to the other pattern. This keeps the body from adapting to and tuning out the patterns.

Functions and indications:

- Function:
  Relieves pain, improves metabolism, improves blood circulation, improves nourishment to tissues, eliminates inflammation.
- Indications:
  Pain, trauma, sprains, arthritis, sciatic pain, facial paralysis, muscle weakness, etc.

Discontinuous/Intermittent wave

A discontinuous or intermittent waveform is basically a dense wave interspersed with a pause. The dense wave fires for about 1.5 seconds then pauses and 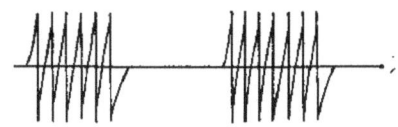 repeats. This is a stronger wave pattern than the previous one, the dense-disperse/sparse waveform.

Functions and indications:

- Function:
  Stimulates the muscles.
- Indication:
  Treats paralysis

How you set these waveform patterns will depend on the machine you use. Let your instructor guide you on this.

This page intentionally left blank.

SECTION 7
Study Guide

Though most of the class this book is designed to accompany is a hands-on class, there is often a written exam that goes along with the skills you are learning and will be asked to demonstrate to show that you know what you're doing.

This section gives you a series of questions and answers to help you study for the written tests you may encounter.

This page intentionally left blank.

Question	Answer
Mugwort/*Artemesia vulgaris* is the herb most commonly used for moxa. What are the properties of this herb?	1. Warm the meridians and expel cold 2. Move qi and blood 3. Open the meridians
When you form a cone from moxa wool there are 3 sizes. What are these 3 sizes?	1. Small – the size of a wheat kernel 2. Medium – bean sized 3. Large – ½ the size of an olive.

Name 5 basic functions and indication for moxa application.	1. Warm meridians and expel wind, cold, and damp
	   a. Wind/Cold Exterior syndrome
	   b. Interior Cold syndrome
	   c. Yang Deficiency
	   d. Bi Syndrome – the W/D/C kind
	2. Regulate Qi and Blood
	   a. Pain
	   b. Skin numbness
	   c. Qi Sinking Syndrome
	   d. Liver Yang Rising
	3. Revive the Yang for resuscitation
	   Yang Collapse Syndrome
	4. Dissipate nodules and remove toxic heat
	   a. Early stage of sore, carbuncle or boil before the pus forms
	   b. Sores, carbuncles or boils that just won't heal after a long time
	5. As a preventative to keep healthy
	   Mostly, scarring moxa on various points, applied yearly.

What are the 4 applications and their functions for moxa sticks?	1. Mild Warming Moxa
	   a. Application: Hold the stick over a point until the skin is pink and warm
	   b. Functions:
	     i. Warm the meridian to expel w/d/c for Bi syndrome (the w/d/c kind)
	     ii. All indications of moxa above, but especially chronic deficient cold diseases.
	2. Circling Moxa

Question	Answer

	a. Application: Move over a larger area in a circular motion or up and down a channel.
	
	b. Function: Warm meridian, circle painful joints due to WDC Bi Syndrome.
	
	3. Sparrow Pecking: move stick rapidly up and down over a single point to alternately warm and cool.
	
	4. Pressing Moxa
	    a. Function:
	        i. Warm the yang and expel cold
	        ii. Move Qi and Blood
	        iii. Open the meridian and stop pain.

What is "direct" moxa?	Can be scarring or non-scarring. Moxa cone is placed directly on the skin (with a thin layer of something to make it stick in place) and lit.
What is "indirect" moxa?	Use of moxa that does not directly touch the skin. This can be moxa cones on top of another medium or any version of moxa that doesn't make contact with the skin.
Why would you use ginger as the intermediary in moxa?	Used for exterior syndromes and deficient cold: common cold, cough, wind/damp Bi, vomiting, abdominal pain, diarrhea. 1. Expel cold 2. Release the exterior 3. Warm the interior 4. Stops vomiting.
Describe the uses of garlic in indirect moxa.	Removes toxins and kills worms. Also good for early stages of carbuncles, sores, boils, insect bites, psoriasis, tuberculosis, scrofula.
Where do you use salt in indirect moxa and why?	Use it at Ren 8, the umbilicus. Two primary uses: • Warm the interior Abdominal pain, pain around the

Question	Answer
	umbilicus, hernia pain, prolonged dysentery, chronic diarrhea, urinary retention.
	• Revive the yang for resuscitation Yang collapse with profuse sweating, cold extremities, hidden pulse.
What about Fu Zi (monkshood) cake for indirect moxa?	This warms the Kidney Yang for yang deficiency problems such as impotence, premature ejaculation, or yin type sores.
What is the Warm Needle technique? Why would you use it?	Using a pre-made moxa needle cone or a hand rolled cone on the handle of an inserted acupuncture needle, then lighting it to warm the needle and transfer the heat into the body. You use this for problems that need both acupuncture and moxa, such as cold damp Bi. Cold Damp Bi symptoms are joint pain, numbness and cold sensations, paralysis, muscle weakness and atrophy. Mainly used locally.
Describe the sensation the patient gets with Moxa.	A warming sensation or slight burning pain. Can be of the local skin, or can be deep inside and/or along the channels.
What areas of application do you do first then later with moxa?	• Yang first, yin last Example: back then abdomen • Upper first, lower later. Examples: heat → body → 4 limbs • Small cones first, big cones later. Fewer first, more later.
How many minutes do you use a moxa stick on an area as a rule of thumb?	10-15 minutes or until the skin turns pink or reddish.
How many moxa cones do you use on a point as a general rule?	3 – 7 or until the skin turns pink or reddish.

Question	Answer
For whom would big moxa cones or a larger volume of cones be appropriate?	Strong people, young men
What areas would be suitable for big/more cones?	Low back, lower abdomen, thick skin, areas of big muscles.
What kinds of diseases would big/more cones be suitable for?	Yang collapse and a severe cold syndrome with a long history.
For whom would you want to use small cones and/or fewer cones?	Women, children, elderly, weak patients
In what areas would you use small cones and fewer cones?	Head, chest, 4 limbs, thin skin, thin muscles.
In what types of disease would you use fewer cones and smaller cones?	W/C/D Bi, upper excess with lower deficiency
What are the precautions you should think about when doing moxa?	1. Explain sensation and possible blister/scars. Have patient sign a consent form. 2. Pick a suitable position for the patient 3. Use cautiously in cases of Yang hyperactivity/yin deficiency, excess heat 4. Stay close to monitor patient's reaction, adjust heat intensity, etc. 5. More attention is required if pt is in coma, has lack of innervation, diabetic, etc.
Where is moxa forbidden for pregnant patients?	Never on abdomen or on lumbosacral areas!
Where should direct/scarring moxa never be used?	Face, private parts, vicinity of large blood vessels, joints.

Question	Answer
How do you treat a burn that results from moxa?	Use a burn cream to stick the moxa cone on and this is a good preventative. You can also apply burn cream as necessary. Infection is the primary concern. • Small burns: can heal by themselves. Use burn cream • Large blisters: puncture with sterile needle, drain, apply sterile gauze • Moderate or severe burns: ER or physician
What are the precautions to give a patient after scarring moxa?	No heavy work, keep local skin clean to avoid infection.
How can you tell high quality Moxa from low quality?	High quality is aged, bluish yellow, very fine, pure (no other stuff mixed in), very soft, and dry. This burns smoother and it's easier to form cones out of it. Low quality stuff is new, blackish brown, has fibers and other stuff mixed in, it's hard and thick and wetter, doesn't cone or burn as well.
What is cupping?	An ancient technique using a cup/jar/horn or something like this, using negative pressure + heat, then placing the cup/etc. over a point. Generally applied to areas of local congestion/stagnation/infection.
What are some general applications for cupping?	• Move Qi and Blood • Expel wind and cold • Dissipate swelling/lumps, clear heat, remove toxins (with bleeding) • Regulates Qi/blood stimulate points.
What are some body type pains you could use cupping for?	Low back pain, stiff neck, shoulder pain, stomachache, abdominal pain, dysmenorrhea, sprains Use on local areas, jiajis, back shus, sacrum.
What kind of Bi syndrome	Wind/damp/cold type arthritis

Question	Answer
could you use cupping for?	Local points or along a whole channel
What kind of respiratory illnesses are suitable for cupping?	Cough, cold, asthma Back of the neck, upper back. Could do specific back shu's or could cover upper back in cups, flash cupping. Sometimes LU 1 and LU 2 if there's enough muscle tissue there.
How do you cup for sores, carbuncles, boils, snakebite etc?	Prick open the sore, apply cup until color of blood changes to normal
How could you use cupping to treat acne?	Not on the local areas, but on Jaiji points. Palpate the points and feel for texture changes in the point. These are reactive points. Cup here.
Where do you cup to treat sunstroke?	Pericardium 3, BL 40, Du14
What is the fire twinkling method of cupping?	Using a cotton ball soaked in 91-95% alcohol held with forceps, inserted into a cup inverted at about 45 degrees to burn the air out and then quickly placing the cup on the point.
What is fire throwing?	You use this on a cup attached to the side of the body (like when the patient is sitting upright). You leave the firey cotton bit inside the cup and attach it to the side of the body. The fuel burns the oxygen out and goes out. Very strong suction. Very hot. Not often used.
What is the cotton attaching method?	Similar to fire throwing. On the lateral side of the body too. Soaked cotton is stuck to the inside of the cup, lit, placed on the side of the body. Hot, strong, not often used.
What is the air pumping type of cupping?	Used with plastic suction type cups. Use an air pump which sucks the air out of the cup. No heat.
When do you use a single	On single acupoints, ashi points, or on

Question	Answer
cup?	disorders in small areas. Du 14 cup might be a good example.
When would multiple cups be appropriate?	Disorders involving bigger areas, whole channels, to regulate the function of several organs, etc.
How long do you retain cups once applied?	Depends. For static cupping or sliding cupping, keep it up 5 – 15 minutes or until skin turns reddish or purplish. (more purple = stagnation). You use less time for big cups and strong suction to avoid the possibility of blistering.
What is flash cupping?	Applying a cup and then immediately removing it. You use this where skin is loose and you can't get good suction. You also use flash cupping for local skin numbness, deficiency, for older people, and for hypo type functioning.
What is sliding cupping and when would you choose this method?	With sliding cupping you use more oil to lubricate the skin where you are going to move the cups. Similar to gua sha. You move the cup back and forth over a large area, over larger muscles, upper/lower back, thighs, etc. Used for pain, muscle tightness, sciatica pain, to expel wind/cold, cough, etc.
How and why do you apply needling cupping?	Needle first, then place a cup that is taller than the needle and apply. Mainly used for WDC Bi syndrome with pain deep inside the muscle or in the bone. This is dangerous any place where there is danger of pneumothorax anyhow.
How do you do blood letting with cupping, why, and when not to?	You bleed first with 3 edged, lancet or plum blossom, then cup over the top of it to suck the blood out. This is good for disorders of Qi and blood stagnation, heat retention. You never do it on big blood vessels as it causes too much bleeding.

Question	Answer
What is the proper way to remove cups?	Gently. You use the tip of a finger to release the suction. Never pull them off forcefully, twist them off, or decrease pressure suddenly.
Describe a good after effect for cupping.	Purple/red spots or bruising that disappears after several days. The more stagnation there is the deeper color the bruises will be. May last up to 10 days on some people. You have to let your patient know beforehand!!!
What *don't* you want to happen during cupping?	What you don't want: blistering. That means either your patient is hypersensitive or you left them on too long. Small blisters will self-resolve after a couple of days. Larger ones should be drained and dressed with sterile gauze to prevent infection.
How do you sterilize glass or porcelain cups?	You can autoclave them or use a chemical disinfectant with double sterilization, especially if there was bleeding.
What if there is bleeding when you cup?	First, use gloves and CNT! Remove the cup slowly to avoid blood spray and hold a paper towel under the cup where gravity dictates the blood will flow when you remove it. Often the blood will congeal, so it is unlikely it will be liquid. Isolate the cups and use double sterilization.
Can you cup very thin/bony patients?	No sliding cupping—too painful. You might be able to cup Du 14. You really want to cup where there is adequate muscle and the skin is elastic.
What about very hairy patients or areas where they happen to have a lot of hair?	No. Sometimes you can use enough oil to make this comfortable, but oil + alcohol + fire + hair? Bad combo.
What precautions should you take with patients who have never had cupping,	Use small cups, less cups, have them lie down, and observe them carefully!

Question	Answer
weak patients, nervous patients, old people, kids…	
List some basic precautions for cupping.	• Check the temperature of the rim and the cup so you don't burn your patient! Don't burn 'em!!! • Short retention during summer or in areas of thinner muscle. • Get 'em comfy first so they don't move around and dislodge a cup.
List 6 contraindications for cupping	1. Not for easy bleeders, leukemia, hemorrhagic purpura, hemophiliacs, blood thinners(?) 2. Contraindicated for severe edema – water will flow to the cupped area 3. No to hypersensitive or non-elastic skin, places with skin wounds, ulcers, tumor areas, hernias, fractures, varicose veins. 4. High fevers, convulsions, non-cooperative or flailing patients 5. Heart beat areas, 5 sense organs, anus 6. Pregnant patients: abdomen or lumbo-sacral area
What are the 3 main types of manipulations for bleeding technique?	• Spot pricking Over a single point (like jing wells) • Scattered/clumpy pricking Prick several times around a diseased area. For sore, sprain, Bi, rash, tinea, etc. Often used with bleeding/cupping. • Blood vessel pricking Prick a superficial vein in cubital fossa like P3 or LU 5, popliteal fossa (BL 40/39), tai yang area, etc.
What are the functions of bleeding technique?	• Clear heat, remove toxins • Remove blood stagnation • Reduce swelling • Open channels, stop pain • Resuscitate

Question	Answer
What are the 5 indications for bleeding?	• Excesses • Heat • Blood stagnation • Pain • Acute disorders

Name 3 precautions for bleeding.	1. Put the patient in a comfortable position (though for BL 40, standing is best)
	2. Apply strict CNT principles.
	   a. Disposable 3 edged needle or lancet
	   b. Wear gloves
	   c. Since you rub the area to get the blood up, clean the points with alcohol afterwards
	   d. Dispose of used needle, cotton balls, etc. in appropriate biohazard containers.
	   e. Wash hands before and after.
	3. Avoid arteries! Veins only.

For whom is bleeding therapy contraindicated?	Weak, aged, anemic, pregnant patients, spontaneous bleeders (hemophiliacs, hemorrhagic purpura, blood thinner patients, etc.)
What is cutaneous needle therapy?	Cutaneous needling is light puncture with a plum blossom or seven star needle hammer. It can be light enough to just redden the skin or hard enough to bring up a little blood. Can be used in a single point or along a channel. Stimulates cutaneous regions of meridians.
For what do you inspect the device before you start?	Examine the needle head to ensure all needles are level, nothing is hooked, broken, no one needle/s is/are sticking out further than the rest. Best to use disposable equipment unless you have access to sterilization equipment.
What is the posture? Where does the force come from?	You hold the hammer at the far end with one fingertip on top of the handle/stem of the hammer. The movement come from the wrist

Question	Answer
	which should be loose and relaxed, but still under control. Grip should be light.
Describe the tapping method.	Use wrist force with a bounding/bouncing tap. You hold the hammer so it is perpendicular to the skin and the whole head hits at once so that no side hits first and penetrates too deeply. Frequency is 70-90/min.
Describe mild stimulation for cutaneous needle therapy, who you use it for, and where.	In mild stimulation you tap just hard enough to turn the skin pink. There should be no pain. This is suitable for weak people, pregnant patients, aged people and kids. It is suitable on the face, head and areas of thin muscle coverage.
Describe moderate stimulation for cutaneous needle therapy and where it is used.	Skin turns to red and there is slight pain, but no bleeding. This is suitable for most cases except on face/head/thin muscle.
Describe strong stimulation for cutaneous needle therapy, who you use it for, and where.	Strong stim involves slight bleeding and pain. It is suitable for those with a strong constitution. You can use it on muscular areas such as shoulder, back, lower back, butt, four limbs where there is good muscle coverage.
Where can you apply this type of technique?	On the back on bladder lines, du channel, jiaji points where the points are reactive. You can tap along the channels below elbow and knee. You can tap single points based on pattern diff. You can also tap local areas for joint disorders, skin disorders (numbness, rash, tinea, psoriasis, alopecia), and in local area for disorders of eyes, nose, face, head, etc.
What precautions must you use for cutaneous needle therapy?	Use CNT procedures! CNT says one device per person...but use common sense beyond this — don't go from fungusy foot to the head with the same device! Use sterile disposables or have access to sterilizing equipment.

Question	Answer
For what is cutaneous needle therapy contraindicated?	Skin wounds, ulcers, scars.
What is Gua Sha? What is it used for?	Gua Sha is applying oil to the skin then using an instrument with a rounded edge held 45° to the skin to rub or scrape the skin. The goal is to raise little "sha spots" similar to the bruising you get in cupping, but likely to be less concentrated. Gua Sha is appropriate for removing blood stagnation, opening channels, removing toxins, clearing heat and regulating the function of internal organs.
What tools do you use for gua sha?	A gua sha plate (or spoon or other tool) and gua sha oil.
What is the difference between direct and indirect gua sha?	Direct gua sha uses oil and direct skin contact. Indirect is no oil and through a silk cloth.

List 4 common indications for Gua Sha.	• External diseases:
	  Common cold, cough, asthma, stomach flu, sunstroke, etc.
	• Pain:
	  Back/shoulder/neck/sciatica pain.
	  Stomach ache, headache, abdominal pain.
	• Gastric problems:
	  Acute gastroenteritis, dysentery, etc.
	• Health preservation:
	  Use lighter stimulation without oil.

List 6 areas where Gua Sha is commonly used.	• Head (yintang, taiyang, GB 20) • Neck (side, GB 20 to 21) • Back (du channel, bladder channel lines, jia ji, above/below scap spine, IC's) • Chest (sternum, IC's) • Four limbs (esp fossas) • Channels and points

Question	Answer
What are the significances of bright red spots after gua sha?	Indicates exterior syndrome, short history, mild illness, good prognosis.
What are the significances of dark red or purple patches or spots left after gua sha?	Can indicate interior syndrome, long history, severe problem or poor prognosis
What are the precautions to consider for Gua Sha therapy?	• Put the patient in a comfortable position, use a clean gua sha instrument, and apply oil before beginning. • The angle should be oblique to avoid cutting the skin. • Strength should be even from beginning to end and only apply one direction (mostly down and out). • Finish one area before moving to another.
How long should you gua sha and what about the intensity?	Gua sha until the spots appear completely. Use lighter stimulation for health preservation, first treatment, aged and weak patients.
How often can a patient get guasha?	Every 3-7 days
What should the patient do for self-care after gua sha?	Rest, drink warm water, no cold showers.
When/where is gua sha contraindicated (4)?	• Never for easy bleeders/hemophiliacs, purpura hemorrhagica, leukemia, etc. • Not where the skin is compromised by wound, rash, sore, scar, mass, infection. • Not on bony areas • Pregnant patients: not on low back, abdomen.
What 3 basic stimulations do you need to know for Electroacupuncture?	• Intensity – how strong stimulation is • Frequency – how far apart each stimulation pulse is

Question	Answer
	• Waveform – shape of wave
What are the 4 very basic steps in e-acupuncture?	1. Inspect the stim machine 2. Insert the needles and manipulate manually to get Qi sensation 3. Hook up the leads to the needles 4. Adjust the stimulation intensity, frequency, and waveform.
What kind of needles do you need to use for e-acu?	Metal handles, thicker needles
What do you do prior to changing/adjusting wave form or frequency?	Turn intensity to off, make adjustments, slowly increase intensity.
What is the appropriate level of intensity for a patient?	Above the sensory threshold and below the pain threshold.
How long do you retain stimulation with this modality?	15-20 minutes.
Which do you connect to the primary point – the negative or positive lead?	The negative lead goes to the primary, the positive to the 2ndary.
How far apart do you place the 2 needles on a circuit?	Not too far, not too close. Too close and you can get cross connect. Too far and you lose sensation. Minimum distance, as a rule of thumb is about 6 cun apart.
What is the frequency, function and/or indication for a Dense Continuous wave?	• Frequency: 50 – 100 pulses per second. • Function: Inhibits sensory and motor nerves • Indication: Relieve pain, tranquilizes the mind, relieves spasms of muscles and blood vessels.
What is the frequency, function, and/or indication	• Frequency: 2-5 pulses/second

Question	Answer
for a Disperse (Sparse) Continuous wave?	• Function: Induces muscle contraction and enhances tension of muscles and ligaments • Indication: Indicated for paralysis, muscle/ligament/joint injury
What is the frequency, function, and indication for a Dense-Disperse/Sparse wave form?	• Frequency: Disperse (slow frequency) and dense (fast frequency) waves alternate, each lasting about 1.5seconds to prevent the body from adapting to a single pattern. • Function: Pain relief, improved metabolism, improved blood circulation, improved tissue nourishment, elimination of inflammation. • Indication: Pain, trauma, sprain, arthritis, sciatica, facial paralysis, weakness of muscles.
What is the frequency, function, and indication for a Discontinuous or Intermittent Wave?	• Frequency: This wave appears on and off rhythmically in 1.5second intervals. • Function: Stimulates muscles • Indication: Paralysis
What are the precautions for electroacupuncture?	• Turn intensity up gradually to avoid strong muscle contraction (needle bend/break/etc) • Never to the level of pain • Mild when near spine or brainstem • Never cross the body's midline with a single circuit • Never for pacemaker/electronic implants patients • Caution for pregnant patients, those with heart disease, seizure patients, aged, weak patients.
What are the advantages of electroacupuncture in disease treatment?	• Better for nerve disorders • Stimulation control ○ More measurable than manual stimulation

Question	Answer
	o Can stimulate multiple points at a time – more than you can squeeze in during a one hour appointment o Can stimulate longer than you can manually with far less tissue damage
How many pairs of points can you e-stim at a time? Bilaterally or unilaterally?	1 – 4. Make sure patient can tolerate well before increasing pairs. Usually unilaterally to avoid crossing midline.

ABOUT THE AUTHOR

Cat Calhoun is a licensed acupuncture practitioner in the State of Texas and soon to be in the State of Florida as well. She attended AOMA Graduate School of Integrative Medicine, earning a Masters degree in Acupuncture and Oriental Medicine. She is passionate about teaching, both formally and informally. Cat has single-handedly created and managed CatsTCMNotes.com since 2008, dispensing notes and clinical pearls to students and practitioners for the past 11 years. She is also passionate about learning, and is currently in love with Master Tung's Acupuncture system.

This book, *Acupuncture Techniques 102: Cupping, Moxibustion, Gua sha, E-Stim, and More*, has a companion book for the 1st half of basic acupuncture techniques in Chinese medicine. Look for *Acupuncture Techniques 101: Safety, CNT, and Needling Techniques* on Amazon. This companion text covers clean needle technique (CNT), safety procedures to keep both you and the client safe, needle manipulation for Qi effect, and needle manipulation for tonification and reduction. Both of these books are vital for framing your understanding of the basic acupuncture treatment methods and safety, critical information you need in order to treat effectively in clinic. Both books are available in digital and print format.

www.ingramcontent.com/pod-product-compliance
Lightning Source LLC
Chambersburg PA
CBHW020908180526
45163CB00007B/2670